PALEO DIET FOR BEGINNERS

Complete Guide for Rapid Weight Loss, Learn How to Lose Weight Fast and Healthy

Adam Peterson

Table Of Contents

Introduction

What is the Paleo diet?

It's a famous dietary plan that is based on different foods just like what had been taken in the Paleolithic era that dates from about 2.5 million - 10,000 years before.

This type of diet generally includes seeds, lean meats, nuts, fish, vegetables, and fruits — foods which might have been obtained by the hunting & gathering in the past. The paleo diet also limits foods which became quite common as farming emerged approximately 10,000 years ago. Those foods are grains, dairy products, and legumes.

There are more names for the paleo diet including Paleolithic diet, caveman diet, Stone Age diet, and hunter-gatherer diet.

Purpose of a Paleo Diet

The main purpose of this diet is actually to return back to the same way of having food that is just like what humans ate at early ages. A paleo diet's main reasoning is a human body is mismatched genetically to the recent diet which emerged with the farming practices — a notion called discordance hypothesis.

Also, farming has changed what human beings ate & established legumes, dairy, and grains like additional staples. It relatively rapid but late alteration in the diet has outpaced people's ability to adapt. So, the mismatch is also considered to be a major contributing element to the commonness of diabetes, obesity, & heart disease in recent times.

Difference between Paleo and Other Diets

Paleo diet is enriched with nuts, vegetables, and fruits— all factors of the healthy diet.

There is a fundamental difference between other healthy diets and paleo diet that is no presence of legumes and whole grains. These are believed to be good sources of vitamins, fiber, & other nutrients. And absent from a paleo diet are all dairy products that are rich sources of calcium and protein.

All these foods are not only good for health but also are more accessible and affordable than foods like nuts, wild game, and grass-fed animals. For a few people, the paleo diet might be quite costly.

Another low carb diet? No, it's not...

What Does Low-Carb actually Mean?

Carbs or carbohydrates are 1 out of 3 primary food types which a human body requires to properly work. The other 2 food types include fat and protein. Carbs provide energy to the body. The human body breaks carbohydrates down for using later or immediately.

When a human body doesn't want to use carbohydrates for the energy purpose as soon as the person eats food, it does store these in the liver and muscles for using later. But, when the body doesn't use the stored carbohydrates, the body actually converts those into fat.

The low-carb diet contains low carbohydrates, usually found in bread, sugary foods, and pasta. Rather, you eat foods like protein, vegetables, and natural fats.

Paleo Diet and Carbs

Paleo diet does call for the followers to actually go back when people were mostly eating food in the Paleolithic era, about 2.6 million years before that is eating as a hunter-gatherer.

Paleo does focus on the high-protein diet along with many fruits and vegetables. Unlike Atkins and keto, a paleo diet is not low-carb; this is due to the foods it actually cuts out, such as grains, processed & refined foods, dairy, and legumes.

Whilst keto does not differentiate between what kinds of fats a person must consume, a paleo diet suggests dieters to not have certain kinds of trans fats and oils.

The primary focus of a paleo diet is to get a person to go back to have food like the hunter-gatherers.

Paleo Permits for Whole-Food Carbohydrates

Though a paleo diet restricts some carbohydrate sources, it is not a low-carb diet necessarily exactly the way keto diet is.

As a paleo diet doesn't force macronutrients, the diet can theoretically be high in carbohydrates, relying on which the foods you eat within certain parameters.

Because legumes, grains, and refined sugars are not allowed, the sources of carbohydrates on a paleo diet are quite limited but aren't eliminated. The paleo still permits carbohydrates from the whole food groups like unrefined sweeteners, fruits, and vegetables.

Conversely, a keto diet does restrict all rich carb sources that include starchy vegetables, sweeteners, most fruits, most legumes, and grains.

Health Benefits of a Paleo Diet

A paleo diet focuses on whole, real, and unprocessed foods. It reduces & mostly eliminates the consumption of artificial sweeteners, preservatives, artificial flavors and colors, additives, hidden sugars, sodium & flavor enhancers. Resultantly, you will eliminate toxins & boost intake of nutrients.

A paleo diet is enriched with nutrients, putting great emphasis on organic fresh fruits and vegetables. Rather than filling up on the processed carbs including pasta and bread, paleo followers can get the dose of goodness on daily basis via organic lean meat, fruits, veggies, berries, seeds, healthy fats, and nuts, all of these are full of minerals and vitamins.

Many people also experience muscle growth and weight loss when eating the paleo diet & keeping their active lifestyle. Enhanced metabolic processes & gut health, stress management, better sleep, a healthy Omega-3/6 fatty acids ratio, and sufficient Vitamin D help in burning the body fat off.

A Paleo diet gives plenty of fiber that together with sufficient water intake & a small amount of sodium intake assist in decreasing the bloat which many people are experiencing on the Western diet. And, Paleo helps in improving the gut flora that is significant in keeping the healthy digestion.

Plus, "hangry" is the combination of angry+hungry that's a common sign for a lot of people who are suffering from chronic or acute hyperglycemia. It also happens if the blood sugar reduces & the person gets hungry soon accompanied by a foggy mind, irritability, disorientation, and fatigue. Meals having fat as well as protein are quite satiating. Also, the energy that the body gets through protein, fat, & glucose from the low GI carbohydrates is released evenly and slowly throughout the whole day. Resultantly, the level of blood sugar stays stable & you do not experience the energy drops quite often; hunger also develops gradually and there are no mood swings.

A paleo diet contains healthy fats which come from seeds, grass-fed meat, nuts, poultry, olive oil, seafood, and coconut. There're not any trans fats. The healthy Omega-3 - Omega-6 fatty acids ratio is also boosted. The correct kinds of fat are vital for decreasing systemic inflammation, maintaining healthy arteries, healthy skin, and brain function.

People who are following the Primal/paleo diet may experience the following benefits:

- Improved sleep
- Mental clarity
- Improvement in people who are suffering anxieties or depression
- Loss in weight
- Lower risk of cancer, heart disease, and diabetes
- Enhanced glucose tolerance; more insulin sensitivity and reduced insulin secretion
- Healthy gut flora
- Decreased allergies

- Improvement in people with respiratory issues like asthma
- More stable and increased energy levels
- Healthier looking hair and clearer skin
- Improved attitude and mood
- No or less bloating, reduced gas
- Muscle growth
- Enhanced fitness
- High immune function & a feeling of well being
- Increased lipid profiles
- A paleo is anti-inflammatory, & many people experience the decrease of pain related to inflammation

What is Better nutrients absorption from the food Involved?

A Paleo diet emphasizes on the unprocessed whole foods, natural sweeteners, plenty of fats such as saturated fat, seeds, grass-fed, nuts, eggs & free-range meat, berries, plenty of seafood and fish, fruits, and vegetables. This excludes legumes, grains, and most dairy & processed sugar. People might include some aged butter and cheese, natural full fat yogurt, healthy dairy foods including kefir, but off-course this really relies on one's sensitivities. A paleo diet also emphasizes on organic, local produce & right farming practices.

There is a general misconception regarding a paleo diet that is it is a low-carb diet along with a huge focus on the meat. Whilst a low amount of carbs might be actually consumed as compare to standard diet via the exclusion of refined sugars and grains, lots of carbohydrates are consumed from nuts, vegetables, and fruits.

There're some hard & fast rules on paleo, but as the paleo diet is a framework & a lifestyle that means several people select to be a bit flexible in this approach that is taking what does work for them & their bodies.

What is In:

- Poultry and meat (that include offal): grass-fed and free-range meat isn't only more ethical and a kinder way for consuming animal products but also it is quite high in the nutrients due to the way animals were raised and fed.
- Seafood and fish: try to select sustainable, seafood and wild fish if possible.
- Eggs: pasture raised and free-range when possible.
- Vegies: starchy and non-starchy tubers & root veggies.
- Berries and fruit: try to stick to the low sugary fruit & berries & just keep high sugary fruit such as mangoes and bananas for days while you want a high carb intake and whenever in season & tasting yummy.
- Seeds and nuts: They're nutritious but several seeds and nuts contain the huge amount of Omega-6 fatty acids that could be pro-inflammatory when consumed in great quantities & if the diet is actually not balanced by the Omega-3 fatty acids in oily fish including sardines and salmon, leafy greens and eggs.
- Herbs and spices
- Salt: try to use a Celtic salt or sea salt to get good minerals.
- Healthy fats: ghee, coconut oil, coconut cream and milk,

- butter (it is mostly fat hence no big issues with lactose), olive oil, duck fat, avocado oil, fish oil, macadamia nut oil, sesame oil and from the grass-fed meats, fish and poultry.
- Condiments: the mustard and high-quality vinegar like aged Balsamic or Apple Cider, pestos and salsas, olive oil, capers, mayonnaise, gherkins, low sugar tomato paste and sauces, olives, anchovies, are all fine, make sure that no nasty preservatives and chemicals are included. Wheat-free soy sauce like Tamari & natural oyster sauce are fine sometimes.
- For baking: chestnut flour, nut meals, sweet potato flour, tapioca & arrowroot flour, coconut flour, use them in moderation because they are either high in carbs or might contain high amounts of Omega-6 fatty acids.

What is Out:

- Grains: particularly wheat & anything with the gluten.
- Legumes: lentils, beans, chickpeas & so on.
- Carbs and refined sugars: fruit juices, bread, sodas, high fructose syrup, white sugar, pasta, artificial sugar, cookies, etc.
- Dairy: particularly milk & low-fat dairy & for people with damaged gluten/lactose or gut intolerances.
- Processed vegetable fats and oils such as kinds of margarine, canola oil (rapeseed), sunflower oil, vegetable oil, soybean oil, & spreads made along with these oils.
- Products that contain Gluten

Fine on occasion:

- All dairy must be mainly avoided, particularly when one is having gut problems & gluten intolerances; however, if you are in good health & do not have sensitivities to the lactose (that is sugar in milk) and casein (that is protein in milk), a bit healthy dairy could go long. Try to not drink cow's milk because this contains high Glycemic Index contrary to yogurt or cheese. Good options are sheep's and goat's milk items, A2 milk of cow & fermented products made with cow's milk such as kefir, ricotta, unsweetened yogurt, butter, aged cheeses, and full-fat cream.

- Natural sweeteners: rice malt syrup, dried fruit, honey, coconut sugar, maple syrup, dark chocolate, molasses for those who avoid fructose.

- Alcohol: dried wines, non-grain spirits.

- Fermented soy like miso, wheat-free soy sauce, and tempeh in fewer amounts.

- Pseudograins such as buckwheat, quinoa, and amaranth are less dangerous but they're great carbs sources & have same anti-nutrients to the grains. These must be carefully prepared to remove the anti-nutrients like phytic acid. Soak these grains in the salted water for up to 8 to 12 hours, wash and cook thoroughly before consuming. Plus, chia seeds fall in the same category.

- Green peas, fresh corn, and green beans fall into legume/grain category but they're ok to use sometimes.

Most Important Rules of Paleo Diet

Could living like some caveman prevent diseases & also make you fit and lean? There are a few doctors who argue that it is the hottest wellness trend nowadays – the paleo. It's one of the healthiest diets. The major key to having primal is about limiting carbohydrates for loading up on organic produce as well as grass-fed meat. When you are willing to go complete steam, the following are a few rules for Paleo.

Make Your Friend Fat

Many diets are quite high in refined grains, carbohydrates, sugar, & industrial vegetable oils, along with a bit healthy animal fats. Yet all cells in the human body contain fat, & we want plenty of nutrient-enriched kind in the animal meat for immune health, hormone balance, & optimal performance. Research reveals that the high-fat diet might cause speedy weight loss and metabolic changes.

Reduce Grains

We have slowly enhanced the consumption of grains with the passage of time. Now, some of the lowest cost & readily available food items are actually made from less costly, subsidized grains including wheat and corn. These foods such as cereal, pizza, bread, and pasta are greatly devoid of the nutrients. These drive up the insulin by putting human bodies in the fat-storing mode, & cause us craving more of those by using the chemical additives.

Consume Nutrient-rich Foods

Vegetables are one of the basic components of a paleo diet and the most nutrient-rich foods. Try to eat the healthiest arugula, kale, spinach, and seaweed. The 2nd most nutrient-rich food is the meat from grass-fed or wild animals such as boar, fish, buffalo, and cattle. Animal meat is very high in omega-3s, B vitamins, amino acids, & other nutrients necessary for good health and wellness of your body.

Feed Gut

Just before refrigeration, the foods were actually preserved by the fermentation, however now, we rarely have fermented foods – & that isn't something very good. Fermented foods have probiotics, the gut bacteria which boost digestion, immune health, and nutrient delivery. Scientists also believe that probiotics in fermented food items such as sauerkraut were vital to the gut health years ago.

Eat naturally raised animals meat.

Research reveals that animal meat from the industrially fed and raised livestock contains dangerous chemical residues & fewer nutrients. Also, meat from the cows which eat high-grains diet is low in omega-3s & CLA. CLA is fat that reduces stomach fat & helps in preventing cancer. For such reasons, consuming wild or naturally raised meat is crucial, as is eating locally grown or organic produce without any genetic modification, fertilizers or pesticides.

Take Little Food Break

The fastest-growing nutrition trend today is IF or intermittent fasting that research reveals helps in reducing the danger of cancer, diabetes, heart disease, and cognitive decline. Some intermittent fasting's biggest proponents include paleo followers. Try to fast for at least sixteen hours several days per week in order to boost mood and energy.

Self-Experimentation

Without mass media, the Internet, and doctors, cavemen had to listen to the bodies in case they did not feel optimal. Everybody is quite different. There are some people who have some trouble with milk products, whilst others cannot eat wheat. One thing is obvious: We might benefit from the experiment. Paleo movement does believe in learning all rhythms of your body & eating & exercising according to how one being an individual thrives best.

Mindset

Lesson No. 1: Perfection isn't a game name.

When you actually get started, there is the delicate balance in order to be stuck between remaining true to your plan and backstroking across the sea of yummy donuts. & for us, a line between them seems almost one millimeter wide.

Might be you are worried that you would slip up ending up in Twilight Zone of the Betty Crocker nightmare, not being able to escape from the vortex of treats that suck you in. Might be you are trying hard enough to exercise the willpower rather than altering a mental framework that you've around nutrition & adjusting the habits accordingly. Eventually, this peters out & leaves you quite exhausted, going towards the phone for ordering takeout again.

Hence, for "staying on the track" you would pour each ounce of your energies into being super perfect. You thrive to stringently stick to the yes and no list of foods for the long time period. You feel guilty or berate yourself while you actually deviate from that list. You also judge the self-worth on how nicely you are eating.

Lesson No. 2: Learn about how food actually affects you.

Now, taking the 1st lesson further, strictly sticking to the yes and no foods list that you read on a site or in some book without even peeking under your "hood" is just like driving your car with closed eyes.

You would get a clear picture of different foods that actually affect you & decide which, in case any food, to not eat for the time long.

More importantly, you can find how the body is basically feeling that is better sleep, stable energy, healthy digestion, good moods, etc.—if you take all the nutrient-poor, overly sugary, processed, and inflammatory foods out which are high in the standard diet. You will give time to yourself for the annoyances to start healing you as you eliminate foods which kept those around.

Feeling better is a pretty good motivation.

You need to follow all of the protocols. If you modify those in order to suit the whims, you might not expect to have the complete benefits. When you do not really alter behaviors for forming new habits then you set up yourself for the regression & "falling the wagon off."

No one has to be stick with the endless unrestricted indulgence cycle that is followed by an ever-present detox or challenge. It is a binge-&-restrict dressed in some different package, & it is quite usual in the paleo community.

Opposite to this, if you make a mindful change then learn how foods can affect you & nourish you with the nutrient-rich food, you'll set up a long-term success. This is easy to navigate the world that is full of sweats and cakes while you know very well that 1) although they might taste good they actually make one feel terrible and 2) you will have this sometimes as some real "treat" then try to be back soon to your regular schedule of the nutritious food.

Plus, you might be putting in your face peppers and tomatoes just to see whether they make the autoimmune condition worst. Or, probably a snack of kombucha and jerky puts the histamine levels on top & you ultimately break out in some skin rashes. For a few people, foods largely encouraged in the paleo just do not work.

It is a great argument for giving attention to biofeedback our bodies provide us.

Lesson No. 3: The Paleo crap foods are yet crap foods, only less crappy.

I am going to come out & say the thing: the paleo junk foods are yet junk foods.

This might not be actually made with similar gluten-containing flour and the hell of sweeteners, more fructose corn syrup, though even if this is made in your home kitchen, this is still a dessert. The treats are quite high in fats.

Also sometimes, you must eat the bread, donut, cake, and cookie rather than the often less satisfying recreation.

Plus, one last point: The ingredients are a bit costly for the paleo junk foods & really do not give similar nutrient density like the staples. In case you are on the budget for money or time, skip the treats and baking.

Lesson No. 4: Eat for helping your training.

While you take a firm decision to hang performance on the paleo framework, this is crucial to intake fat, protein, and carbohydrate to help above-normal output & repair any wear-&-tear that your body's going through. What is more, biasing all of the choices towards the most nutrient-rich foods possible most of the time would make the strong foundation of your health to assist your performance.

When the frequency of your training is a bit high (think for many days or several sessions per day) or the training is a bit challenging, having protein & glucose-based carbs (such as starch and starchy vegetables) for the post-workout would assist you in getting a huge jump on the recovery.

Lesson No. 5: It isn't just all about food.

Whilst food is the vital component of your lifelong health, this isn't the only one. To focus on healthy food at the cost of exercise, sleep, & managing stress is also doing yourself the disservice.

Plus, when attempting to have a handle on these things could be a bit overwhelming, making little alterations over time does add up. Remember, there is a big difference between perfection and discipline. Would you've time where sleep actually goes down, you cannot go to the gymnasium, & your life is quite stressful? Yeah, but surely that does not represent every single day of you for months & years.

Take-away action: You can evaluate how good you are staying active, sleeping, & dealing with tensions. In case you want to make some changes, make your targets small as well as manageable. Find different ways to make yourself accountable, like writing in some journal and/or having a good buddy. You could do it. You could make changes.

Getting Started: Most Import thing is your mindset

1. Do not jump in at once.

2. Try to phase out every food group (legumes, sugars, beans, dairy, and wheat).

3. Just jump in, & cut the bad stuff out. (Thirty Day Challenge is very good to do it.)

4. Take one garbage bag, & clean your kitchen out.

5. Begin with making the snacks paleo, and then dinner, lunch, and breakfast. Or just change one meal per week.

6. Skip a non-paleo product from the diet at one time.

7. Slow transition by no more purchasing bad stuff & eating what is left in the house until it's all gone.

8. Conduct deep research.

9. Read about paleo solutions.

10. Know the 1st stage is all about detoxing.

11. Do not be much strict at the start.

12. Plan every meal for the very first 2 weeks.

13. Get your entire family on board.

14. Plus, do a 7-day juice fasting to skip previous cravings & withdrawal signs.

Mindset

15. Do not refer to this as the 'diet'.

16. Rather than thinking regarding how large a change this is, try to pay attention to the reward the change would bring.

17. Do not even begin cheating (as cheating could get out of your control).

18. When you fall the wagon off, jump back on.

19. Must know that you'll fall off your wagon.

20. Do not keep eating food which is made to be just like the things you cannot have such as desserts. This approach will not help you in changing your lifestyle.

21. Keep in mind it gets simpler and easier.

22. Know it is your lifestyle and not your diet.

23. Do not make this harder than it's.

24. Try to keep sight of a large picture.

25. Must hang in over there.

Make the Paleo Simple and Easy

26. Buy a fridge so you could stock meat in large quantity during sales season.

27. Make some boiled eggs for the quick breakfast meal.

28. While at weekends, plan the meals, & prepare sufficient food that can last all week.

29. Find some go to snacks for while you are hungry but not have time to cook food.

30. Make your snacks before time.

31. Plan in advance.

32. Pack your food while you are leaving your house.

33. Keep this as simple as possible.

34. Eggs, vegetables, and meat.

35. Plan 2 meals ahead hence you will get all of the ingredients that

you might want on hand.

36. Know very well while to cheat for avoiding falling off your wagon.

37. Keep the list of all foods on your fridge, & use this one as the list of different options while you need to have snacks.

38. Stay from the desserts away.

39. Delete all takeaway contact numbers from the smartphone.

40. Eat the way which suits you and not the way somebody else thinks that you must eat.

41. When you are having some hard time eating hundred percent paleo, use the organic sprouted grains bread & grass-fed butter.

42. In case, you have ever seen this advertised on your TV, do not eat this.

43. Remain hydrated by drinking water in large quantity.

44. Make double or big batches of the food, & use all leftovers for the next meal.

Enjoying Paleo Fun

45. Lots of ham and bacon.

46. Make your own paleo ketchup.

47. Eat dark chocolate and bacon in moderate quantities for giving up the junk food easily.

48. Have some cheat days as well.

49. Snack on nut butter, almonds, and healthy nuts.

50. When you've your sweet tooth as well, find recipes of healthy paleo desserts.

51. Use all fresh herbs.

52. Find the paleo versions of all recipes that you can make.

53. Find recipes which you love.

54. And, tweak the recipes for making those suit you.

Also, probably the most crucial one:

55. Just do this.

Paleo and Weight Loss

Could a Paleo diet assist you in losing weight?

A paleo diet is the most famous diet around.

This contains unprocessed, whole foods & emulates how the hunter-gatherers used to eat.

Every advocate of the paleo diet believes it could decrease several risks of modern health problems, pointing out the hunter-gathers who didn't face the similar diseases which people nowadays do, like obesity, heart disease, and diabetes.

In fact, several studies reveal that by following the paleo diet might lead to weight loss & main health improvements.

What's a Paleo diet?

A paleo diet boosts eating unprocessed, whole animal & plant foods such as nuts, meat, seeds, fish, fruits, eggs, and vegetables.

This also avoids the processed foods, grains, sugar, and dairy though some of the alternatives of a paleo diet allow options including rice and dairy.

Contrary to most diets, the paleo diet doesn't involve any counting calories. Rather, this restricts some food groups that are the main sources of calories.

Research reveals that those diets which emphasize the whole foods are far better for the weight loss & overall health. They're much more filling, contain fewer calories & decrease the processed foods intake that are attached to several diseases.

A paleo diet does imitate the hunter-gatherer diet & aims to decrease the risks of different diseases. This promotes eating unprocessed, whole foods & restricts foods such as grains, dairy, sugar, & processed foods.

Five Ways the Paleo Diet Might Assist You in Weight Loss

A paleo diet could help you in losing weight in several ways. Following are five of them.

1. Low in Carbohydrates

Decreasing your carbohydrates intake is the best way to lose weight. More than twenty-three studies reveal that the low-carb diet is quite effective rather than low-fat and traditional diets in weight loss.

The paleo diet reduces your carbohydrate intake by removing usual sources of carbohydrates like potatoes, bread, and rice.

This is vital to note that carbohydrates are not bad necessarily for you; however, restricting the carb intake could decrease the daily calorie intake & help you in weight loss.

2. High in Proteins

It is one of the most significant nutrients for your weight loss.

This could enhance your metabolism, decrease the appetite, & control many hormones which regulate the weight.

The paleo diet encourages eating protein-dense foods such as eggs, lean meats, and fish.

In fact, an average paleo diet gives between 25 to 35 percent calories from the protein intake.

3. Decreases Calorie Intake

For the weight loss, you generally have to decrease the calorie intake.

That is why this is crucial to select those foods which are filling because they could fend off your hunger & assist you in eating less.

When you are struggling with your hunger, the paleo diet can be perfect for you because it's incredibly filling.

Several studies have revealed that a paleo diet is quite filling rather than many other famous diets such as diabetes & Mediterranean diets.

Moreover, studies show that the paleo diet can help you in producing more hormones which do not keep you hungry after the meal, like GLP-1, GIP, and PYY as compared to the diets that are based on the traditional guidelines.

4. Removes Processed Foods

Most modern diets are the main cause of why obesity is increasing day by day.

This does encourage eating processed foods that are full of calories, less in nutrients, & might enhance the risk of several diseases.

Several studies reveal that the rise in intake of processed foods actually mirrors an increase in obesity.

A paleo diet restricts all processed foods because they weren't there during the Paleolithic time.

Rather, this encourages drinking fresh fruits, lean sources of protein,

& veggies & healthy fats that are low in calories & nutrient enriched.

5. Removes Added Sugar

Such as processed foods, eating much of added sugar might be dangerous to the weight loss efforts as well as health.

This adds a large amount of calories to your food & is lower in nutrients. Also, a huge intake of the added sugar can boost the risk of diabetes and heart disease.

A paleo diet removes added sugar totally and rather boosts natural sources of the sugar from vegetables and fresh fruits.

Although vegetables and fruits have all natural sugars, they give many necessary nutrients such as water, vitamins, and fiber; all of these are good for your health.

Research Reveals It Assist You in Weight Lose

A lot of studies suggest that the paleo diet is quite impactful for weight loss.

In a study, fourteen medical students were asked to follow the paleo diet for 3 weeks.

And during the study, the students lost the average of about 5.1 pounds (or 2.3 kg) & decreased the waist circumference about 0.6 inches (or 1.5 cm).

Some studies compared a paleo diet & low-fat diets. They have revealed that a paleo diet is quite effective in losing weight, even with the same calorie intakes.

In research, seventy obese ladies aged sixty and above followed either the paleo diet or the high-fiber, low-fat diet for twenty-four months. Obese women on a paleo diet actually lost weight about 2.5 times more after 6 months & 2 times more after 1 year.

By the 2-year mark, both of the groups regained weight a bit, but paleo diet group had lost almost 1.6 times more.

One more study showed thirteen individuals having type 2 diabetes. They followed the paleo diet & then the diabetes diet (moderate-to-higher carb and low-fat) over 2 consecutive 3-month time periods.

And, on average, people following the paleo diet actually lost 3 kg (6.6 pounds) & 4 cm (1.6 inches) more from the waistlines as compared to the group that is doing diabetes diet.

Unluckily, most studies on a paleo diet are fairly new. So, there is very less published research work on long-run effects.

It is important to note that a few pieces of research on a paleo diet do comparison its impact on weight loss with the other diets' impacts on the weight loss. Whilst studies show that a paleo diet is far superior.

Paleo boosts many Other Health Aspects

Along with paleo's effects on the weight loss, this diet is also linked to a lot of health advantages.

Might Decrease Belly Fat

Your belly fat is quite unhealthy & enhances the risk of heart disease, diabetes, and other health conditions as well.

Studies revealed that a paleo diet is good at decreasing the belly fat.

In a study, ten healthy ladies followed the paleo for 5 weeks. And, on average, these women experienced an 8-cm (3-inch) reduction in the waist circumference, that's an indicator of the belly fat, & around a 4.6-kg (10-pound) weight loss.

Can Decrease Blood Sugar and Raise Insulin Sensitivity

The insulin sensitivity does refer to how your cells actually give a response to insulin.

The boost of insulin sensitivity is an amazing thing because this makes a human body quite efficient at eliminating sugar from the blood.

Research has shown that a paleo diet enhances insulin sensitivity & reduces blood sugar.

In the 2-week research, twenty-four obese people along with the type 2 diabetes had followed either the paleo diet or the diet with legumes, moderate salt, whole grains, & low-fat dairy.

Both of the groups experienced enhanced insulin sensitivity, however, the impact was much strong in the paleo diet group.

Can Lower Risk Factors of Heart Disease

The paleo diet is just similar to the diets that are recommended to boost heart health.

This is quite low in the salt & does encourage the vegetables, lean sources of protein, fresh fruits, and healthy fats.

That is why it is not a coincidence that research has proved that the paleo diet might lower the risk factors of heart disease such as:

- Triglycerides: many studies shown that following the paleo

- diet can lower blood triglycerides about 44 percent.
- Blood pressure: The analysis of 4 studies containing 159 people revealed that the paleo diet decreased systolic blood pressure up to 3.64 mmHg & diastolic blood pressure up to 2.48 mmHg.
- LDL cholesterol: Many studies found that following the paleo diet can lower "bad" LDL cholesterol up to 36 percent.

Might Lower Inflammation

As inflammation is the natural process so it assists your body to heal & fight different infections.

But, chronic inflammation is detrimental and could enhance the risk of different diseases such as diabetes and heart disease.

A paleo diet also emphasizes some foods which could help in reducing the chronic inflammation.

This promotes eating vegetables and fresh fruits that are good sources of several antioxidants. Antioxidants assist bind & neutralize the free radicals in your body which damage the cells in chronic inflammation.

A paleo diet recommends eating fish because it is a great source of proteins. Fish is enriched with omega-3 fatty acids that might lower chronic inflammation via suppressing hormones which promote inflammation like IL-6, TNF-α, and IL-1.

Tips to Increase Weight Loss by the Paleo Diet

When you would like to follow the paleo diet, the following are some useful tips to assist you in losing your weight:

- Eat a lot of vegetables: They contain fewer calories & have fiber, assisting you to stay full for the whole day.
- Eat different fruits: Fruits are nutritious & incredibly filling. Try to eat 2 to 5 pieces each day.
- Make ahead: Avoid temptation by making some meals ahead to assist you through your working days.
- Have plenty of sleep: Your night's sleep could help you in burning fats by keeping the fat-burning hormones regular.
- Remain active: Regular exercises help in burning extra calories in order to enhance weight loss.

How to start?

This could take some accommodation and preparation. Whilst eating grass-fed red meat and oil is acceptable & healthy on the paleo diet, consuming fats is the major hurdle several low-fat dieters actually fight to control. There're so many oils which aren't friendly to a paleo diet. While starting, try to remain stick to lard, coconut oil, tallow, olive oil, and ghee (clarified butter).

Where to begin?

Starting your new eating plan might seem a bit daunting. For avoiding feeling overwhelmed, you can have a meal plan that will be perfect for the first week!

On the time crunch? You can use a day for preparing all the food for your busy week. It would make sure the week worth of healthy eating.

Following is the collection of a fast meal and snack ideas. Here is how to make snacks and meals and which are quick.

Yummy Fast Paleo Snacks, Breakfasts, Lunches, and Dinners

Delightful Snacks are:

- Deviled guacamole eggs (cut in half the boiled eggs, remove the egg yolks, combine egg yolks & guacamole in the mixing bowl, fill the egg whites & sprinkle with the seasoning of your choice!)
- Macadamia nuts (one oz.)
- Fat bombs
- Cherry tomatoes and olives
- Diced vegetables with the guacamole
- Almond butter and celery
- Deli turkey & sliced cucumber along with the paleo Mayonnaise
- Scotch Eggs (boiled eggs and wrapped in the sausage)

Fast Breakfasts:

- Breakfast muffins (pumpkin muffins)
- Hard-boiled one dozen eggs, pour 2 to 3 in the container & you are set for the whole week.
- Chorizo Sweet Potatoes Hash
- Quick Breads
- Bake one pound of the nitrite-free bacon.

- Smoothie: Coconut milk, almond butter, fruit (vegetables), plenty of ice cubes.

Quick Lunches:

- Leftovers
- One big salad along with olive oil, meat, seeds or nuts, avocado, lemon juice or vinegar, hard-boiled eggs, and vegetables. Keep the seeds or nuts separate thus they can stay crunchy!
- Cabbage Apple Slaw and grilled protein
- Use one leaf of the lettuce for filling with the sandwich.
- Raw vegetables with one can of tuna.

Dinners (which make large portions hence one has last night's leftovers for the next week):

- Eggs and bacon (Who does not love this breakfast for the dinner?) You could always fry a few turnips (or some sweet potatoes) & onions as the good substitute for some hash browns.
- Turn the grill on. Vegetables & any type of meat are just ultimate in the paleo, & yummy after being cooked!!! Add some paleo-friendly oil if necessary.
- Acorn Squash along with Beef and Cauliflower Rice
- A stew of the leftovers (fat or oil of your choice, leftover or browned meat & onions, a stock or broth, veggies that you want to use, spices, & simmer)

- Brown meat & vegetables with garlic, chili powder, salt, & crushed red pepper; pour on greens for the "taco salad" along with salsa.
- Chicken Zoodle-cine Alfredo- chicken breast, noodles or zoodles made with zucchini & a mandolin spiralizer or slicer, & Cauliflower Alfredo Sauce

How much weight loss is good?

It is usual for anybody attempting to their lose weight and want to lose this very quickly. However, evidence reveals that those who lose their weight gradually & steadily (almost one to two pounds each week) are succeeded at keeping the weight off. A healthy loss in weight is not just about a "program" or "diet". It is all about the ongoing lifestyle which includes the long-term alterations in daily exercise and eating habits.

When you have got the healthy weight then by depending on the healthful eating & physical activities during the whole week (almost 60 to 90 minutes of moderate intensity), you're successful at maintaining your weight off.

Macro counting

What're Macros?

It is the short form for macronutrient, & refers to 3 large groups of the food nutrients that are:

- Carbs
- Proteins
- Fats

Macros differ from micros that refer to small groups of the nutrients including vitamins, amino acids, and minerals.

Several people know the idea of a low carbs diet, where the carbs are decreased to the low percentage of diet intake. Nowadays, tracking the macros is about more than carbs.

While somebody is tracking the macros, they are paying some attention to the number of grams of fats, carbs, and proteins that they are eating. Usually, the main target is to maintain each one within some certain amount of a day's overall food.

How Counting Carbohydrates & Macros Is Same

- Both need a food tracking journal or app to record per day's entire food intake.
- These require awareness of what someone is having versus just winging this.

Counting Macros

- Macros permit great customization of the diet.
- Macros give a wide variety of advantages; for instance, bodybuilders and athletes who do not need calorie restrictions could benefit from just tracking how much macronutrients they are taking in or achieving a healthy balance of the nutrients.
- Macros are also applicable to each and every one.
- Macros are quite effective as compared to calories for producing the results that you want.

Macros are a bit different method of measuring the food intake which completely takes into account the value of separate nutrients as compared to simply counting calories.

How to Measure the Macros?

For measuring the macros, you need to have a clear notion of the calories that you want each day to get your aim. Whilst this is not a strict calorie counting, this provides you the strong baseline to begin with. For the average weight woman who is average height, about 1,800 - 2,000 calories per day will be appropriate. For loss in weight, 1,500 - 1,800 calories can be quite suitable.

For measuring your macros, all you need is to have a clear notion about the calories that you need a day to get your goals.

You need to keep this in your mind that the macro tracking is individual, & there's not 1-size-fits-all which works. The calorie baseline has to take all of the following points into consideration:

- One's height
- One's age
- One's activity level
- One' current weight
- One's situation (for instance, postpartum, pregnant, premenopausal, breastfeeding, attempting to conceive)

For instance, in case you are a healthy weight female who is not pregnant & who works out on daily basis, you are going to get more calories as compared to an overweight female who is not active.

To have a clear notion of how much amount of calories you want per day, & how this translates into your macros, you might use an online

calculator or you might calculate all the calculations, as follows:
The following calculations are tailored for females.

10 into weight (kilogram) + 6.25 into height (centimeters) – 5 into age (in years) + 5 = daily caloric baseline

Then, you have to take into consideration the activity level; as if you are active then you burn calories more than the calorie baseline.

Light activity: Calorie baseline into 1.4

High activity: Calorie baseline into 1.8

Sedentary: Calorie baseline into 1.2

Moderate activity: Calorie baseline into 1.6

In the above example, a five foot three inches, 140-pounds, the forty-year-old female who got light activity will need one baseline of about 1,783 calories per day to keep her recent weight. To lose, she'll have to decrease calories by fifteen percent or change the ratios of macronutrient for reducing carbs & prioritize protein.

Let us say, although, that the woman needs to maintain the weight. So, breaking down 1,783 per day calories into macronutrients is the best done by using the online calculator, however, you have to know well about what your macro targets may be. The below-mentioned section would assist you in narrowing the main focus on what macronutrient range can work for you in the best possible way.

You cannot follow somebody else's macronutrient plan. You have to customize this to work perfectly for you relying on the individual variables. Within these calculations, there is still some space for tweaking or flexibility, but it's a good one to begin.

Five Reasons to Calculate Your Macros

If you want to lose your weight or not, be mindful of your macronutrients ratio that you are eating could take your health and diet goals farther as compared to flying blind. Following are 5 purposes why you may need to track the macros, & the basic guidelines to start.

1. Weight Loss

Macronutrient priority: 45 percent protein, 25 percent carbs, 30 percent fat

Whilst it isn't true for everybody, the majority of individuals who want to lose their weight are not getting much protein at their breakfast & they're eating many carbohydrates. Focusing on the protein spread daily would assist to maintain blood sugar level and limiting carbs would prevent the fats storage from excess carbohydrate intake.

Do not fear fats for weight loss. It is selecting fat quality which matters, hence opting for 30% fat from good sources such as pastured eggs, salmon, grass-fed meats, olive oil, avocados, coconut oil, & the like would give better results as compared to limiting the fat & eating more junky or refined carbohydrates.

2. Autoimmunity/Thyroid Health

Macronutrient priority: 40 percent fat, 30 percent protein, 30 percent carbohydrates

Many people who have autoimmune or thyroid issues might also want to lose their weight. But in such case, it is good to lose the weight & equip your body to heal. Excellent fat is also nourishing for autoimmune and chronic conditions, & slightly more carbohydrates might be essential to enhance energy level in the face of the thyroid or depressed immune system.

3. Strength Training

Macronutrient priority: 40 percent protein, 35 percent fat, 25 percent carbs

Whilst most females are not targeting to get ripped, the athletic females who do the CrossFit and lift weights may have to pay attention to enhancing the muscle tone. It's typically accomplished with the low carbs diet & consuming a bit more protein rather than fats. Still, while this comes to making muscle definition and being the high performing athlete, kind of activity & individual body might need more macro customizing.

4. Menopause

Macronutrient priority: 35 percent protein, 35 percent fat, 30 percent carbs

Females who have experienced the hormonal shift which is menopause might find their body actually responds quite differently to foods than this did before the menopause. The fairly balanced macronutrient plan for such phase of your life might be quite effective at maintaining weight balanced and hormones as well, although females might still want to customize the ratios relying on the activity level, health factors, & food sensitivities.

Macronutrient counting is for serving your health needs & may have to be actually adjusted relying on several seasons of your life. Tracking the macros in the food journal app, keeps many things easy and simple.

5. Fertility

Macronutrient priority: 45 percent fat, 30 percent carbs, 25 percent protein

Females who need to become pregnant & grow their baby healthy want fat. They do not have to be fat, however true, fertility is actually based on the optimized hormones, & fat assists hormones to communicate properly. Fertility fats cannot come from the old thing, and have to be basically sourced from the good quality, paleo fats such as coconut oil, avocados, tallow, grass-fed beef, lard, pastured eggs, olive oil, and salmon.

Fertility carbohydrates also relying on good quality must be typically sourced from the high fiber veggies & fruits, & must steer clear of the refined grains, products, and sugars.

Get Healthy using Paleo methods

A paleo or Paleolithic diet for short is famous as gluten-free diet along with the main attention to having food like our ancestors ate food: it includes seeds, lean meats, nuts, fish, vegetables, and fruits. It's a totally gluten-free and dairy-free diet which doesn't need calorie portioning or counting, so it's great for busy persons on the go. The Mayo Clinic stated that following a paleo diet has shown to give the below-mentioned health benefits:

- Enhanced glucose tolerance
- Low triglycerides
- Weight loss
- Good blood pressure control
- Good appetite management

Fats

Not clear about Omega-6and Omega-3? Confused about what "good fat" is or what does make them "good"? Sick of listening about the grams of this & grams of that even without some reference to the foods that you eat? Following are a few quick facts for setting the record quite straight, do not need any biochemistry degree!

Kinds of Fats

There're 3 main kinds of fat: polyunsaturated, saturated, and monounsaturated. The major differences need to do with the chemical structure.

- Saturated fat is the paleo-friendly – no, this does not give you cancer, or heart disease, or diabetes, or something else.
- Polyunsaturated fat is more complex. It has got 2 types: Omega-3and Omega-6. Without even going too much into details, just aim to actually limit the Omega-6 & get Omega-3 more.
- Monounsaturated fat is paleo-approved as well.

Sources of Food of the Paleo Fats

On the paleo diet, fat must be the main source of calories (energy). This will not make fat. In fact, it is more likely to assist you in getting (or staying) thin, as it is quite satisfying, burning fuel source. Fats from the whole foods should not be ignored: keep the egg yolks, and a chicken with skin on, & cook with the real butter!

Fats You Need to Avoid

All types of fats are not good! You must aim to actually limit the Omega-6 polyunsaturated fat. The below-mentioned foods would set you up for much Omega-6 hence avoid those:
- Margarine and "buttery spread," to name a few. Real butter is healthy for you but fake butter isn't good.
- Industrial seed oils: soybean oil, canola oil, peanut oil, corn oil, "vegetable oil" (can be all or any of the previous).
- An excessive amount of seeds or nuts. It is good to eat these; just keep this to almost a handful daily.

How Much of Fat Must I Eat?

For people who actually understand that having fat intake does not make fat, it is a bit scary to dive headfirst into "demon nutrient" of the previous 2 decades. Is this really alright to make the soup by using coconut milk – does not that have much of the fat? Is this really alright to cook food with one whole tbs. of butter? For eating the egg yolks? For leaving chicken with skin on?

Yeah! This really is alright! In fact, it is far better than just alright; it is great for you. While you switch to the paleo diet, you are cutting out all unhealthy junk items, but also the source of grains or calories. You have also got to get calories from elsewhere, & fat is actually where it as at.

Even without involving into the calorie-counting (that is not essential or recommended on the paleo diet), here're some tips for ensuring that you are eating much of healthy fats:

1, Do not make much effort to discard fat from the whole foods. Leave the skin on the poultry. In case, you are going to add dairy in the Paleo menu then make this full-fat dairy. Cook your omelets along with whole eggs and not only the yolks.

2. Ensure each and every meal contains one of the below:

- At least two tablespoons of cooking fat (for example, coconut oil)
- A serving of fats (for example, coconut milk or avocado), or
- A fatty animal food (for example, fatty ground beef, pork belly, bacon)

For instance, in case you're having a salad along with tuna (that is lean), and throw in avocado, and use dressing with olive oil. It is fine to match and mix, and it is also nice to consume more; it's a minimum.

3. You also need to avoid including the extreme or excessive amount of fats in the meals. Do shots of the olive oil, and also you can deep-fry your food. But it is not a big issue when you are eating the whole foods. It is pretty tough to overeat fats from the whole food sources as many people stop wanting this after some time.

In addition to this, as far as you entirely free yourself from the fear of fats "making you look fat," the taste buds & hunger would guide you for an appropriate amount of fats intake.

Mistakes to Avoid for Beginners

For the beginners, here is a detailed explanation of 2 general beginner hang-ups regarding fat, & how to not have them:

Trap No. 1: Protein Not/Overload Enough Fats

It's what happens to ninety percent of those who try to do paleo diet without allowing to go of the low-fat dogma first. It is also called "Faileo."

Breakfast: apple and egg white omelet.

Lunch: skinless grilled chicken breast with the salad and a tiny drop of olive oil.

Dinner: broccoli and steamed tilapia.

Often the menu is a prelude to different questions such as "why I'm constantly quite hungry?" & "where did my energy actually go?"

You must know how a person is cutting sources of natural fats from the whole foods (by using just skinless chicken breast and egg whites), limiting the salad dressing (one "little dab" of the olive oil), & going out of the way to select cooking techniques like steaming and grilling that do not involve fats.

Trap No. 2: Not Enough of Food

The person, in this case, is consuming fatty foods; however, she is so feared of having "too many fats" which she is eating an insufficient amount of those. The menu will look just like:

Breakfast: Two boiled eggs.

Lunch: Half cup of the soup that is made with the leftover chicken & coconut milk; the carrot sticks. Five tablespoons of mayonnaise.

Dinner: Two rashers of the bacon and roasted cauliflower.

Fats as the calorie percentage are perfectly fine; however, it's the meal plan for one ant!

Carbohydrates

Though the paleo diet restricts some carbohydrate sources, this is not essentially a low-carbohydrate diet just like the keto diet is.

As the paleo diet doesn't force macronutrients, the diet can be theoretically high in carbohydrates, relying on which food items you select to consume within the particular parameters.

Because legumes, grains, and refined sugars are not allowed, the carbohydrate sources on a paleo diet are quite limited but not removed. paleo allows carbohydrates from the whole foods groups just like fruits, veggies, & unrefined sweeteners.

Opposite to this, the keto restricts rich sources of carbs that include starchy vegetables, most legumes, most fruits, sweeteners, and grains.

Because of the fact total carbohydrate intake should remain quite below a specific threshold to keep ketosis, several high-carbohydrate foods, regardless of sources, simply do not fit into the keto diet.

Protein

Protein is a main part of this diet industry. It is married to the similar low-fats dogma which brought obesity epidemic in a prominent place, main weight-loss programs cannot recommend the diet that relies on fats. With the increasing popularity of low-carbohydrate diets for weight loss, carbs have become the black sheep that leave proteins as the "good" macro.

The paleo dieters, luckily, are not interested in mainstreaming the nutritional guidelines. Good animal fat is the major part of the Paleo meal plan: also much-demonized saturated fats are nothing to be feared of. However, it does not mean that the Paleo diet eliminates other important macronutrients – carbs are the most debated topic, everybody agrees that the healthy diet also includes some protein.

What's Protein?

Proteins are complicated polymers (molecules) that are formed from small subunits known as amino acids. All of the twenty well-known amino acids belong to 1 of 3 groups. The very first group, known as essential amino acids, does include the10 amino acids which your body can't make itself; you need to get much of those in the diet. And, in the 2nd group, nonessential amino acids that include amino acids which you could synthesize from the essential amino acids and from the protein. Regardless of their name, the amino acids are not less important as compared to the essential cousins. These may not be actually "essential" for getting in your diet, but they are yet "essential" from the body's viewpoint. The 3rd group, conditional amino acids, has those amino acids which are typically nonessential, however, become essential while the body is under strain (for instance, in case you are not well).

Protein also plays an important role in your body. It is a primary building block that functions as a structural "skeleton" for the cells. Several kinds of proteins perform a large number of different functions like enzymes (substances which drive biochemical reactions such as digestion) are one kind of protein, the other proteins assist cells in the body to communicate, & motor proteins are for different large-scale movements such as muscle contraction and microscopic movements that are involved in the cell reproduction. Also, proteins assist in transporting the substances within your body, & could combine to make sophisticated mechanisms.

Make sure to have all ten essential amino acids on a daily basis sounds like one tiny chore, but luckily its answer is quite simple: you need to eat meat. Any type of animal products (like dairy, meat, and eggs) is the "complete protein," means that it has all essential amino acids, hence on the paleo diet, to get amino acids in should not be an issue. People who worry about matching as well as mixing particular sources of protein are usually vegetarians, as plant proteins such as beans are usually not complete.

The Macronutrient Ratios and Goldilocks: How Much Amount is Right for You?

Protein indisputably does play a crucial role in all physical processes, & unlike glucose (that your body might synthesize in case you are not eating carbs), you cannot manufacture proteins from any other source. When you do not eat essential amino acids then your body would begin breaking the muscles down in order to get these. In other words, the healthy diet wants enough protein, preferably complete proteins that are found in the animal products.

Also, at the low limit, the diet containing 10 percent protein by the caloric intake would meet all essential requirements. Eating less than ten percent protein for the extended time period risks deficiencies in essential amino acids. And, on the paleo diet, consuming less than 10 percent protein is a bit tough – you will need to make serious efforts to restrict the meat intake & take just the fattiest cuts.

Ten percent can be actually considered as the low end of a healthy variety of protein intake. The "high-protein diet" also has 20 to 29 percent protein, whilst a "very high-protein diet" contains 30 to 39 percent protein. An ability of a person's body to metabolize the protein ends at 35 percent. So, "high protein" is basically the relative term: advocates of the higher protein intake aren't claiming that this must account for the major amount of calories.

These ratios rely on a normal (almost about 2,000-calories) diet. An absolute amount of the protein is significant. At its upper limit, the protein toxicity starts to set in while you consume above 920 calories (230 grams) of protein per day (note that it isn't the similar thing as consuming 920 calories meat, as some calories in the meat come from fats). On the 2,000-calorie diet, nine-hundred and twenty calories are 46 percent of the energy achieved from protein, above "very high protein" ratio. On the 5,000-calorie diet, 920 calories toxic level is just 18 percent of energy. It does mean that on the higher calorie diet, a protein percentage should be lower to remain within the healthy range.

The calculations also leave us with the fairly large variety of protein consumption – 10 percent to 35 percent of the diet, as far as protein doesn't consist more than total 920 calories. A person can survive on every protein intake within the given range, however, that doesn't mean the maximum protein consumption is quite broad. Primitive hunter-gatherer diets give a clue about how much proteins the humans are equipped to manage. Loren Cordain reveals that the hunter-gatherers ate about19 to 35 percent of the energy as protein, it's actually the overestimation as Cordain bases calculations on an "average" animal while, traditional hunter-gatherers singled out the fat animals for consumption in the herd. Most of the hunter-gatherers ate closer to 10 to 20 percent of calories. Hence, for the people having no particular nutritional considerations, 10 to 20 percent protein is the appropriate starting point.

The Risk of Additional Protein

Continuously consuming inadequate protein (below than 10 percent) would cause some serious issues, however, in reality, this does not happen quite often. Particularly on the paleo diet, many people face a few issues eating adequate protein. One more general issue is consuming too much. Relatively higher protein diet (20 to 29 percent protein) may not be good, but this probably will not do some major damage, especially when you consume that protein with the high-quality fat & carbs. Some people caught in the trap of attempting to have large percentages of the energy from sources of protein, particularly after cutting their carbs consumption if they stop consuming grains.

In several cases, the protein's overconsumption is simply because of the lingering fear of fats –restricting carbs isn't actually alien to the mainstream diet suggestion, but when you're raised to review that the "low-fat" was actually synonymous with the "good for you," to embrace the butter as the healthy food could be a bit challenging. People stumble at the very first by attempting to consume the "less-fat paleo" diet that ends up being the high-protein, as if you are restricting carbs & fats, protein is the main source of energy left. Such type of diet can easily have 60 to 70 percent of calories such as protein – the meal of chicken breast without skin or tuna along with veggies does not give much of carbs or fat.

Firstly, such a diet might make keeping the caloric deficit quite painless: as protein is a satiating macronutrient, consuming plenty of protein assists you to stop feeling hungry. The sating effect does not last long – as in the short run, the high-protein diet might assist you in feeling full whilst in the caloric deficit, however, in the long term, your body would adjust. Such an extreme addition of protein could lead to the entire variety of health issues.

Plus, protein toxicity is the general term which refers to dangerous effects of consuming much of protein. This is caused due to the amount of protein that is in the diet, & by the protein ratio to other macros (carbs & fat). If you break protein down into energy, your kidneys first have to remove the nitrogen from amino acids, the process is known as deamination. The process increases a chemical known as ammonia as the byproduct. As ammonia is quite toxic so your liver can convert this into a product that is urea. Urea passes out of your body via urine. Consuming a high amount of protein could also put unnecessary strain on the liver & kidneys because they try to convert protein into the useful energy form.

Processing of ammonia properly needs carbs & fat like co-factors, hence the protein overload without other 2 macros is very stressful. It's why the lean protein is satiating – the body knows that this can just digest the small amount; you can feel full soon. Fatty meats are less satiating as your body contains enough co-factors (fats) to process the protein.

When you just consume protein even without accompanying fats or carbohydrates, not only would you overwork the kidneys and liver, but also you will not get enough fat-soluble micronutrients which your body wants for other vital processes. Some health issues that actually result from such type of protein that is overload are typically well documented. Inuit referred to the toxicity of protein as the "rabbit starvation," it is not because this results from consuming "rabbit food" in huge amount in raw veggies form, but because Inuit actually suffered from this while the only item they might get was the rabbit, that is lean meat. Signs of the "rabbit starvation" include weight loss, weakness, & a common feeling of illness. Additional protein intake might lead to anxiety and mood problems, by interfering along with the neurotransmitters functions in the human brain.

Whilst overload of the dietary protein might cause some serious issues, periodic protein restrictions – the same as intermittent fasting – could be quite advantageous. Restriction of intermittent protein assists your cells in performing a type of "spring cleaning" of useless and old proteins which will otherwise gather in the body. The process is known as autophagy; it is one of the advantages of the intermittent fasting, however, for a specific perk, you do not necessarily need to abstain from the food. Restriction of protein alone (when consuming as many fats & carbs as you want) would give the same outcome.

Takeaway: Protein for the Paleo Diet

To claim that a specific percentage of a diet must be protein is quite interesting scientifically, but such type of recommendation isn't applicable directly to the way many people think about the food. They do not purchase "thirty-six grams of protein;" rather they purchase half dozen of eggs or one salmon piece. Weighing & measuring each and everything that you eat is just an option, however, this could be a bit time-consuming as well as often impractical. Luckily, it is not essential. Most people might make a rough estimate about how much food they are hungry for; so doing the similar for protein is not tough.

Generally, to remain within the range of protein intake, just try to pay attention to the fat as it is the main calories source (but not the major part of the diet in terms of volume). Do not consume protein without fats – have fatty cuts of the meat as pork shoulder & lamb,

& eat chicken along with its skin. There is nothing wrong with the lean meats such as tuna, but consume these along with another source of fat, like delicious avocados with tuna steak.

Whole foods

When you think about organic groceries then Whole Foods is the very first store which comes to your mind – this is a retail giant that contains natural foods. Whole Foods also carry plenty of the paleo staples, including wild-caught seafood, grass-fed meat, & one complete line of the grain-free flours. This has some items which look like paleo but are not.

Primarily, the paleo diet meal plan is based on the whole-food nutrients sources.

The whole food is typically a food which has also undergone a minimum processing amount by the time this gets to a plate.

A paleo diet encourages removing all of the ultra-processed foods & replacing these with the whole foods including nuts, fresh vegetables, fish, and meat.

It is particularly evident along with the exception of processed oils, fats, & sweeteners in paleo's "rule books."

Most Common Mistakes

Low-carbohydrate diets are all the rage recently, & the paleo is also no exception. Relying on how the Paleolithic ancestors might have consumed, the paleo meal plan includes those foods which they will have hunted as well as gathered. The followers of a paleo diet actually stick to oils, meats, seeds, fish, nuts, fruits, and vegetables. They avoid starchy vegetables, sugar, grains, dairy, legumes, and beans. Though the paleo sounds quite promising, individuals do make plenty of mistakes while consuming this way. The paleo diet mistakes can hurt than helping their health.

Studies are mixed on the efficacy, but a paleo diet's benefits are blood pressure control, weight loss, and low blood sugar & triglycerides. Because this is a quite restrictive diet, the nutrient imbalance can occur based on how you are eating. When you take a decision about hopping on a paleo trend then make sure that you are doing this right. Following are the paleo mistakes that you might be making & how to avoid these.

Depending on the Packaged Food Items

On the traditional paleo diet, you are supposed to not eat all processed foods. However, as the paleo diet has now become popular, many packaged products contain a paleo label. If some food product says 'paleo' does not make this healthy food. The paleo cookies are cookies. Eat them sometimes, but make sure to prepare yours with the whole-food items.

You aren't Consuming Enough Calcium.

This sounds just like the argument that some ill-informed nutritionist will make like to why the paleo diet is not healthy; however, there is some truth about it as well if you think the way many individuals follow what they actually consider to be the paleo diet.

Also, you do not want dairy in order to get adequate calcium for good health. There're several calcium-enriched foods which adhere to the paleo standards.

The issue is many calcium-dense foods which are permitted on the paleo diet aren't ones which you might be eating properly.

For the health nutritionists ask you to have things like nuts, bone-in fish, leafy greens, and bone broth, the truth is many individuals aren't including them on daily basis to get daily calcium requirements.

If you consider the store-bought almond milk provides you the essential calcium that you need then understand one thing that the kind of calcium which these items are actually fortified with (that does not naturally contain) is the kind of calcium which is tough to absorb, & these products generally do not include fat-soluble vitamins K2, A, and D that help in regulating calcium absorption & metabolism.

You need to get six-hundred mg of calcium daily from the sources of whole foods. Try to reintroduce the full fat, grass-fed dairy in case you have not yet, as it is a good calcium source if well tolerated. It could be kefir, cheese, fluid milk, and yogurt when you feel great drinking this. You may even need to try raw milk.

Do not be afraid of the dairy product just because many Paleo dieters say it is a no-no. There're so many people who actually do great on dairy & you may be one of those.

Not Consuming Adequate Fiber

As, legumes and whole grains are actually off-limits on a paleo diet so most people do not eat enough of fiber. This nutrient is crucial, as it might assist with maintenance of weight, low cholesterol levels, and stabilized blood sugars. Within a paleo diet, sources of fiber include seeds, fruits, nuts, and vegetables.

Consuming Excessive Meat

You necessarily have not to be the vegetarian in order to live a healthy life. But consuming meat at each meal might not be a very good habit for a body, A person who follows a paleo diet must think about the meat as an accompaniment than the main. At every meal, eating 8 ounces of meat is way too much. This might put unnecessary strain on the liver and kidneys. To avoid the biggest paleo mistake, make a balanced plate which includes healthy fat and non-starchy veggies.

Having Wrong Sources of the Saturated Fat

Every fat is not created equal. There's a large difference between eating 2 servings of the nuts every day as compared to consuming salami & cured meats on a daily basis. Also, the standard Western diet is actually abundant in the lab-made saturated fat. For somebody who is transitioning from the Western diet to a paleo diet, there is risk involved that there's confusion about the health advantages of fats. The processed meats are not basically paleo-approved. Thus, stick to the plant-based fat sources with the grass-fed & sustainably sourced meat.

Avoiding Carbs for No Apparent Reason

It's the number one problem that is seen in those patients who are actually struggling hard on a paleo diet. Most people who begin paleo are usually drawn for easy and quick weight loss whilst consuming low-carb foods such as bacon, prime rib, and avocado.

Several paleo bloggers suggest limiting fruit, minimizing the starchy veggies, entirely avoiding the sweeteners, & keeping carb consumption low to increase weight loss. And most paleo recipes creators actually default to the low carb recipes, even when they do not mean to.

There is a wrong belief that carbs are detrimental for every individual: because they cause cognitive decline, premature aging, fat gain, & cancer. Such belief is adequate to scare people away from every type of carb, even those which come in the healthy whole foods such as starchy veggies as well as fruits.

Whilst a low carb diet could be therapeutic for some people, like those having severe digestive disorders, diseases, or diabetes which affect the cognitive function, there're several people who are following the low-carb type of paleo just because they believe that there is no need for carbs & that eating carbs would lead to dangerous health outcomes. Most people are highly active & struggling to do high-intensity exercises nearly on a daily basis. It isn't a healthy combination.

Carbs aren't toxic while metabolized normally. Whilst they might be good in treating specific conditions, they are not the main cause of these conditions. And, limiting those can assist people in weight loss so they do not cause weight gain in healthy individuals. For some people, a reintroduction of carbs even assists in increasing weight loss if combined with suitable caloric intake & physical activities.

Some knowledgeable paleo dietitians suggest that people who do not have issues with increased blood sugar might do themselves some harm by limiting carbs excessively. Females might be prone to the problem of insufficient carb intake. Most paleo dietitians tell that there might be benefits of having the "higher" carb diet.

Ultimately, individuals vary largely on their carb needs & tolerance. When you're feeling lethargic or moody, gaining weight, & generally feeling not well on the low carb paleo diet then you might find that increasing your overall carb intake enhances the symptoms which you have developed because of following the inappropriate low-carb diet.

It's about more than what you actually eat

The paleo is an amazing holistic lifestyle which contains nutrition and other factors like sleep and exercise. In case, we do not recognize sleep being a main component of the good health, we're missing a significant ingredient. Plus, sleep helps with stress, weight, and hormone & metabolism regulation.

Avoiding fat

It's time to avoid every fat phobia. There is evidence relying on the research which reveals that quality fats such as avocado, nut butter, nuts, flaxseeds, olives, and coconut oil that improve hormones, nourish brain, & help with insulin sensitivity. More sugar would drive your cholesterol more than some avocado ever can.

Approaching this like some healthy detox

Consider paleo as putting so much nice which you forget about processed, unhealthy, and high sugar foods of the previous time period. This form of nourishment would let you rid toxins when you move quite close to the foods which aren't full of colors, chemicals, & additives.

No planning

Yeah, like anything you're good at, planning the new paleo diet would take time as well as planning, but soon it'll become a habit & you wouldn't think about anymore. So, take your time to find easy and yummy recipe ideas like this & plan your shopping lists and meals.

Portion distortion

Many people get fat as they move to the paleo lifestyle. Any food in huge excess, whether nutritious or not, a huge amount of calories are there. Due to foods like oil, nuts, and coconut butter are on a paleo list of healthy foods that does not mean you'd consume them in large quantity.

Paleo is not about everything or nothing

There're a lot of versions of the paleo diet based on whose blog or book you are reading. Just follow its top rules: getting rid of additional sugars, removing processed foods, decreasing vegetable oils, and eliminating gluten will assist you in achieving better health. So, find what does work for you and not what somebody has told you to consume, but what makes the body to feel good.

Not a discernible shopper

If the label shows 'gluten-free,' it does not mean that it's really healthy. Become the label reader & if you can't pronounce its ingredients & your grandmom would not recognize a word then step away.

Not having a large variety in carbohydrates

No, a sweet potato is not the only Carbohydrate out there! Zucchini, broccoli, & other green vegetables are great sources of carbohydrates. Eating different vegetables in the paleo diet is essential for the synergy of minerals, vitamins, & enzymes for the healthy body cells & a good digestive system.

Thinking Paleo is the weight loss program

As you know that paleo is the healthy lifestyle & if you're having a diet that is full of unprocessed, whole, and clean foods then you would gain energy as well as vitality. Whilst the paleo lifestyle isn't some weight loss program rather the principles of clean eating that it espouses might ultimately lead to weight loss.

Consuming Natural Sugar in Abundance

The natural food, a paleo nutrition meal plan removes processed & genetically modified types of sugar; however, the general meal plans allow coconut nectar, fruit, and honey. These're natural sweeteners that give great benefits. However, they have many drawbacks as well. The higher fructose element in the sweeteners might put some burden on your liver & hamper the ability of detoxification. This can result in adrenal issues and hormonal challenges.

The natural sugars also give fuel for all unwanted microorganisms like parasites and yeast. As the microorganisms can take control over in the gut that they would release endotoxins which inflame your body.

They'll develop gut inflammation which damages your intestinal membrane setting for the leaky gut syndrome. It might affect your sex hormones and adrenals that will cause energy issues & hormonal imbalances.

Decreasing sugar by reducing the intake of maple syrup, honey, coconut sugar, etc. is critical boosting hormonal control, energy, digestive function, and liver detoxification. Stay away from the high sugary fruits like pineapple, bananas, and melon & stick with fewer quantities of low-glycemic fruits including lemons, berries, limes, and grapefruit. Limit yourself with famous nut and fruit bars as they might be convenient. However, they have so much fructose which would disturb the hormone balance.

Consuming Nuts in Huge Quantity

The primal/paleo nutrition plan removes the use of grains & decreases starchy carb intake. As you look elsewhere for getting your calories, the nuts are a simple solution. You are familiar with the nuts as most people eat nuts daily throughout their lives & they're easy to buy in any store.

Almond flour is very famous non-starchy flour that is an alternative for the baking purposes. Many people crave baked items & they end up using large amounts of the flour for various muffins, pies, bread, and pastries that they make. A paleo diet does not generally put any restrictions on the nuts amount consumed daily.

Anti-Nutrient Content in the Nuts

Nuts might be hazardous if they are consumed in huge amounts. Nuts have phytic acids which bind to all major minerals such as magnesium, zinc, and calcium. The huge amount of phytates in the diet could cause mineral deficiencies. All of these minerals are vital for hormonal balance and energy production.

There're enzyme inhibitors that are present in the nuts which block the normal enzyme activities in your body. It might lead to energy problems and digestive challenges. Sprouting or soaking seeds and nuts helps in reducing phytate & enzyme inhibitor counts & thus makes the seeds and nuts more bioavailable.

Many seeds and nuts are high in omega 6. Many people are in the dominance of omega-6. Taking more and more omega 6 only increases this imbalance & causes chronic inflammation.

Hence, taking in fewer omega-6 dense seeds and nuts such as sunflower seeds, almonds, pecans, and cashews will be healthy for you. They can focus on the high omega 3 in pumpkin seeds, walnuts, flax, hemp, and chia.

Consuming seeds and nuts, in moderation, could be helpful for your health. Eating not more than half a cup of the almond flour per week or two cups of nuts is fine.

Avoid Grass-Fed and Raw Dairy

Many people who are following the primal or paleo nutrition plan have taken dairy products out of the diet. Though, it's a good step for some period of time. No one must be eating typical grain-fed and processed dairy which is the Western cuisine staple. Such kind of dairy is so much inflammatory as it's filled with omega 6, antibiotics, pesticides, and hormones.

The only form of dairy which is 100 percent grass-fed dairy is in raw form. Good kinds of dairy are Amasai & fermented whey items, raw fermented goat, kefir, cow or sheep cheese, and yogurt.

Grass-fed ghee or butter is free of casein because it's just milk fat & contains no protein hence it is a healthy food to have. On an autoimmune nutrition plan, you can use ghee.

Eating Wrong Veggies

Broccoli is a good paleo vegetable. Vegetable intake is surely encouraged on a paleo diet, however, there're some veggies which are off the limits.

Snow peas, string beans, edamame, and green beans are on the veggies to not eat list as they're considered legumes, & those who observe the diet believe that there are detrimental health effects linked with these.

Given that there're several other paleo-friendly vegetables to select from, it is typically an easy diet mistake to correct.

You're not getting enough manganese, magnesium, and selenium.

Almonds are a healthy magnesium source. paleo eliminates legumes dense in minerals such as manganese, magnesium, and selenium. Hence, it is best to add a lot of replacements into the diet. In order to make sure that you are having adequate magnesium in the diet, it is great to consume magnesium-dense foods including avocado, spinach, and almonds often. Selenium is also found in sardines, nuts, and tuna. Manganese is typically found in leafy veggies and nuts.

You're making the Paleo meal too bland.

Consuming paleo does not mean that you have to consume bland food. There're many sauces that you could make which are paleo-friendly. It includes the red curry coconut sauce that is made with the coconut milk, lime juice, red curry paste, a small pinch of fish sauce, & coconut aminos. Pesto could be easily made paleo-friendly, making the dairy-free Italian classic with toasted almonds, basil, olive oil, hemp seeds, salt, garlic, and lemon juice.

You did not clean your pantry out.

Set specific shelves for your paleo-approved foods. The main paleo mistake that you might be making isn't cleaning your pantry out & accidentally consuming foods which aren't considered paleo. One more benefit of cleaning your pantry out is you always look at the foods which you might include in the diet, vs. being reminded of those foods that you're no more able to eat.

You are not checking fluid intake.

There're so many paleo-friendly fluids which have caffeine. Whilst you might have various food choices, do not forget to see the drink choices. And, artificially-sweetened energy drinks and soft drinks like red bull and diet coke aren't included. Rather, try drinking paleo-friendly beverages that include black coffee, lots of water, and green tea.

Avoiding Food Quality

Quality of food is a major premise of a paleo diet. For most people, it's an afterthought and just a consideration. For example, take a lettuce-wrapped big mac than one grass-fed burger. Such foods have a similar amount of fat, protein, and carbs. By a few definitions, they're equally 'paleo'. Both of these meals contain disparate metabolic outcomes. The main focus of a paleo diet is macronutrients quality than their ratio.

Conventionally the raised animal items & pesticide-laden produce would not contain successful results. They might be an ok place to begin. The GMOs, antibiotics, herbicides, steroids, pesticides, hormones, and some other chemicals would continuously wreak the long-run havoc on the metabolism. Make sure to buy high-quality protein and organic produce (grass-fed lamb and beef, wild game & fish, & pasture-raised pork and chicken), & fat (unrefined organic olive oil, grass-fed ghee, expeller-pressed organic coconut oil, pasture-raised lard, and grass-fed butter) whenever possible.

In case, eating everything organic isn't financially easy for you then you need to start where you might. Although all organic foods would yield fast outcomes, the whole foods diet of all types is yet a good place to begin.

Paleo is More Than Just A Diet

There are a lot of people who actually hear the term 'diet' & their efforts as well as thoughts immediately stop along with the food. The paleo is basically more about a lifestyle rather than just some food-based diet. The food also plays an important role, but in case you do not get succeeded in addressing all other aspects of a complementary lifestyle of the paleo diet, you would not experience the whole potential of this program.

Whilst you entirely commit to a paleo diet then it is crucial to take the hard look at the other elements which allowed the ancient man to survive.

- **Sleeping**

You need to make this sure that you prioritize about 7 to 9 hours of your sleep time at night regularly. Even a night of insufficient sleep might disrupt the regulation of your blood sugar that will ultimately make you stressed, possibly to have processed carbohydrates, & cranky.

- **Sun Light**

People have actually evolved having a close link with nature than just sitting inside the home all day long. If you do not expose to the sunlight then your health might suffer. You should try to go outside of your home for some exposure to the sunshine for about 30 to 60 minutes per day with naked skin.

- **Stress & Play**

Fun activates your parasympathetic and 'rest & digest' branch of your nervous system. It is quite often ignored in the high-stressed world these days. Try to create some stress management protocol which fits into the life & make enough time to actually escape from stress every day. You can dance, breathe deeply, go out with your friends, meditate, watch entertaining YouTube videos, & do not take life so much seriously.

- **Movement**

Professionals are calling a sedentary lifestyle and sitting the new smoking. Also, movement on a daily basis is essential as your body is created to move & functions best whenever movement is actually incorporated into the lifestyle. Try to find an exercise that you love & incorporate this for about half an hour each day five times every week. Even the brief twenty-minute walk gives you a good outcome.

You are Behaving Too Tough

Yeah, there's such thing as becoming so much concerned with the diet, & it is unluckily far too usual in the paleo group.

There are some experts who call this orthorexia. While others quite bravely admit using paleo as the cover-up for all eating disorders. There are a few people who just turn their blind eye, and call this discipline. Some individuals even think that they are struggling hard with the diet as they are not much restrictive. It might not be actually farther from reality.

There are some people who are on an autoimmune protocol despite never having some autoimmune disease. Some females also follow a very low carb diet, likely overexercising, chronically undereating, & dealing with long-run amenorrhea. Several people literally think about the food all day long that they get distracted from some other important stuff of life because of their obsession with the food.

Unluckily, it is quite common, particularly in the modern age of information that is overload as everybody has his own thinking about what is the best diet to have. (As if the "perfect" diet actually exists for everybody).

It does not mean that you should stop thinking about following principles of your diet & simply eat Frosted Flakes and Big Macs. However, you should consider the strictness of the diet & whether it is at an essential level for you or not.

Many people absolutely should avoid specific foods relying on the current situation of their health. Though, putting oneself on the overly strict diet even without having any strong reason to do this is no more than a recipe for some disaster. Whether such disaster manifests as anxiety, weight gain, depression, increased G.I., distress or some other kind of detrimental side effects which come from excessive and inappropriate food restrictions that you might bet it would show up at any point.

There are plenty of people who have a perfect deal of benefits from the reintroducing a large variety of foods that are back into the diet. Yes, this also includes specific non-paleo foods such as sweeteners, dairy products, & even properly cooked wheat and grains products.

In case you have been consuming a super strict paleo diet & you are not able to articulate the conditions why you are doing so then you might have to think about loosening up a bit. Life is actually short & enjoying the food & not stressing regarding your paleo diet on a daily basis must be your main target, even if you're not feeling good. You could eat healthy and quality food & still enjoy the meals, & mental health & happiness must be the top priority.

Supplementation

Supplementation or no supplementation?

To make a long story summary, for many people, nutritional supplementation might be essential for optimizing health as well as performance. So, SAD or Standard American Diet has also left so many people with much of specific nutrients & a bit to no other sources.

Most importantly, due to destructive agricultural practices and bad soil quality, the foods aren't as much nutritious as they were used to be. It is still one more reason why local, grass-fed and free-range products are the best.

Other Reasons for Supplementing might be Essential

- More exposure to the toxins
- A rise in lifestyle as well as environmental stress
- Less exposure to the sun (because of being inside all day)
- A diversity of the plants
- More use of birth control and antibiotics (liver damage)
- Bad sleep quality
- Standard American Diet or SAD focus on the processed foods which damage your enzyme production and stomach acids & make difficulty in the absorption of nutrient

In case you have continuously taken the paleo approach about nutrition then you are consuming some of the high nutrient-rich foods available & assisting the body to survive.

While comparing your day of paleo intake to your day on the Standard American Diet, it is pretty obvious that quality of the calories eaten on the paleo diet is so good than those found in the standard western diet.

It is good news as you need the majority of nutrients in the diet to come from the food you eat. The human body is made to retrieve & break down different nutrients from the whole foods. "The American Journal of Clinical Nutrition" has published a paper in which it stressed the significance of getting your minerals as well as vitamins from the food.

This particularly highlighted the following:

- Free radicles are decreased by eating brassica veggies.
- Consumption of tomatoes has a huge impact on prostate tissue as compared to an equal amount of lycopene.

Only Take one Multivitamin a day, Right?

Most people take one multivitamin each day and they believe that they're giving protection to themselves from diseases and chronic health issues. But, studies reveal that many multivitamins give very little advantage at all and specifically while this comes to reducing the risk of chronic health problems like:

- Cardiovascular disease
- Cancer
- Heart attacks

Several multivitamins use the synthetic substitutes to the whole food minerals and vitamins (these are called "isolates"). The body might just absorb the tiny amount of these isolates & it might utilize less than that.

Multivitamins & taking a pill each day has now become quite famous as they are more convenient. In case, you are searching for some good multivitamin then try to avoid the Walgreens, Walmarts, CVS, & Targets. Rather, look for the labels which show the following:

- Quality control
- NSF or ISO certified
- Natural
- No allergens or additives

There are many good multis that would display such things on the label prominently.

Now, with this, the most population doesn't want many nutrients which are there in the multivitamins. Several multis would either provide you more of specific nutrients rather than you actually want (for instance, B6), & not others which are tough to have enough of through the diet (for instance, magnesium).

Also, most of the nutritional requirements could be achieved by just taking some selected vitamins because they are which most of the population is actually lacking.

When you actually need to learn which minerals as well as vitamins you require, you should have done the nutritional testing hence you are then able to find out what really you want.

Omega 3 (DHA/EPA)

The SAD or Standard American Diet mostly emphasizes on Omega

6 fats that are found in the industrial processed seed oils & animals that are fed grains, soy, and corn. It has also contributed to Omega 3 to Omega 6 ratio of about 20:1. Plus, a good ratio of the Omega 6 to the Omega 3 will be pretty close to 6:1.

And, these poorly-fed animals and oils are very much inflammatory & importantly lead to several other modern ailments and diseases in the world.

Krill oil and fish are pretty much high in the Omega 3 fats &, more importantly, enriched in DHA as well as EPA – 2 significant fatty acids essential for your brain functioning. By supplementing along with the Omega 3 fatty acids & avoiding all industrial seed oils, you might balance out the Omega 6 - Omega 3 ratio.

Plus, taking roughly 1 to 2 tablespoons of oil of fish each day would probably be more than enough assisting to balance these ratios out if you are eating the paleo foods most of the time.

Based on how much active you're, how much sleep you're getting, what is your body size, & how good the diet is, you might have to consume more, however, for now, these 1 to 2 tablespoons of fish oil will do the trick. Choose for a liquid version than capsules as liquid versions are easier to absorb, do not have artificial ingredients, & stay fresher.

Advantages of taking the fish oil on a regular basis include:

- Enhanced fat burning
- Decreased risk of heart disease
- Decreased risk of diabetes

- Enhanced metabolism
- Higher insulin resistance
- Decreased risk of cancer
- Less joint pain

That is only the tip of an iceberg. There've been several studies that reveal other advantages too.

There are few high-quality brands there which make bad tasting fish oil. But, in case you just cannot have this for some reason then you should try your best to eat about one pound of the wild-caught salmon each week. It must provide some of the similar advantages.

This must be actually noted that when you are having blood thinners, you can experience some bleeding disorder, and are going to have some surgery, so fish oil must be avoided because it might tend to thin the blood out a bit.

Also, you might enhance the Omega-3s level in the paleo diet by not eating soy, grain-fed animals, and corn, & by consuming more grass-fed meat like lamb and beef or the wild-caught seafood such as salmon instead.

Good sources of Omega 3:

- Whole foods – wild-caught seafood, grass-fed beef, and lamb
- Amount – two to five grams of DHA or EPA
- Supplement – krill oil (much stable as compared to fish oil)

Vitamin D

Typically, vitamin D is fortified or included to those foods that are in D2 form that is almost 87 percent less potent as compared to vitamin

D3. It is also converted by your body to the active form quite slowly, & has a bit short shelf life rather than D3.

And, vitamin D3 is pro-hormone that is important for physiological function and immunity. This also enhances the glutathione levels – an antioxidant that is very essential for detoxifying your body of the heavy metals.

Some Other Advantages Include:

- Strong bones by the calcium absorption
- Assists with osteoporosis
- Tight junctions in the gut (for avoiding leaky gut)
- Fights stress and depression
- Decreases risks of cancer

D3 is easier to have, only if you make some concerted efforts. Expose your face, arms, neck, and legs to the sunshine & eating wild-caught seafood such as Wild Channel Catfish and sockeye salmon are perfect ways to become close to 2,000 to 5,000 IU of the vitamin D which are suggested on daily basis.

Best Sources:

- Supplementation – Cod liver oil
- Whole foods – Organ meats, wild-caught fish (sardines, salmon, tuna, mackerel), egg yolks, and raw milk
- Amounts – 2,000 - 5,000 IU each day (some suggestions quote about 1,000 IU for 25 pounds of a body weight who aren't exposed to sun quite often)

Probiotics

Most modern diseases which plague our society start from the stomach. That's why consuming foods that enhance gut health might make a big difference to your long- and short-term health.

- Chrohn's Disease
- Arthritis
- Depression
- Irritable Bowel Syndrome
- Celiac Disease
- ADHA

They are just a few recent autoimmune-related health problems which could be improved in case suitable gut health is well maintained.

Because of a rise in the use of antibiotics, NSAIDs (Advil), & the intake of processed foods & industrial seed oils (like cottonseed, soybean, to name a few) inflammations in the body & especially in your digestive tract has become quite common.

Your liver assists to get rid your body of the toxins that help in reducing inflammation. However, with a low level of the good bacteria in your body, elimination system of the body (skin, bowels, and bladder) could get all the clogged up that makes it tough to eliminate some toxins.

Also, good bacteria may create such condition in which minerals, B-vitamins, & other nutrients could thrive. The bacteria in your body break down cholesterol and lipids. This does strengthen the gut/brain connection, assisting to decrease the risk of behavioral health issues that include anxiety, autism, and depression.

Best Sources:

- Supplementation – Sedona labs iflora Multi-Probiotic Powder
- Whole foods – Kombucha, sauerkraut, kimchi, and kefir
- Amount – Ten million CFU or colony forming units each day through probiotics, enhancing your dose every 2 to 3 weeks by almost ten million CFU until fifty million CFUs are actually taken per day

Magnesium

It is a quite tough nutrient in order to get much of via your routine diet alone (and even when you're a pro at having the paleo). It is also one of the main reasons that supplementing the regular paleo diet can make a big difference to health.

Magnesium assists with sleep, blood clotting, muscle contraction, energy production, & a whole host of important bodily functions such as the development of the new cells. This is good for:

- Cramps
- Headaches
- Heart arrhythmia

You might have the deficiency of magnesium in case you got weakness, experience fatigue or chronic headaches, or loss of your appetite.

Best Sources:

- Supplementation – Natural Calm (that is drinkable)
- Whole foods – Avocado, spinach, pumpkin seeds, Swiss chard, and raw almonds
- Amount – Eight milligrams before going to bed (don't take along with the D3 as both compete for the absorption)

Other Vital Supplements

K2: added calcium might be actually deposited in your arteries (that is calcification). In order to avoid it, vitamin K2 helps calcium metabolism. Also, K2 aids in preventing heart disease.

- Whole foods – Raw grass-fed hard cheeses, natto, grass-fed beef, organ meats (liver), and egg yolk
- Amount – Hundred mcg per day

Vitamin A (Retinol): Assists in assimilating water-soluble minerals, vitamins, & proteins. This is a very strong antioxidant.

- Whole food – Liver (organ meats)
- Supplementation – Cod liver oil
- Amount – 10 to 15,000 IU from the cod liver oil

Selenium: Assists in strengthening your immune system, improving thyroid function, and fighting cancer

- Whole foods – Wild-caught tuna, Brazil nuts, and oysters
- Amount – Two-hundred mcg per day

Vitamin C: Assists to maintain a high level of strong antioxidant in your body, glutathione, & fights infection. This also aids with connective tissue as well as collagen production.

- Supplementation – Garden Of Life Raw C, one-hundred percent acerola powder
- Whole foods – Red peppers and acerola cherries
- Amount – Five-hundred mg to one gram per day (more when fighting some infections)

Iodine: Assists in promoting thyroid function properly
- Whole foods – Eggs, sea veggies, raw milk, and spirulina
- Supplementation – Potassium iodine capsules
- Amount – one mg per day

Simply for reminding you, the supplements are a good method to "supplement" well-balanced and healthy diet in order to increase mineral and vitamin consumption & to decrease inflammation & risk of serious diseases.

The supplementation is mentioned in this book in which most people are deficient in due to the food eaten on the SAD. In case, you're interested in searching out the nutrients that you specifically require then kindly consult a doctor or naturopath for the nutrient test.

Supplementation for Specific Conditions

Above-mentioned are a few supplements which might be quite helpful to big chunks of people. There're some individual conditions where this can be suitable to take the supplement as, for a particular condition or other that is you cannot have that specific nutrient from your food.

- People who are recovering from the malabsorptive diseases such as Crohn's Disease might find some supplements of

- different nutrients.
- Individuals who cannot consume a specific food group due to some reason can use a supplement for the nutrient that they cannot get otherwise.
- After the bariatric surgery, a lot of people have to use supplements throughout their whole lives as they are no more capable of absorbing particular vitamins.

They're all types of main reasons why particular supplements can be good for you; the main point is to choose those deliberately.

You must define what you actually need & find proof that the particular supplement actually fulfills that requirement.

Opting Supplements Carefully

Many people think that supplements need to pass a type of safety testing just before they visit the market. That is not true at all. There's no federal regulation about supplementation before people hit the supplements shelves. Its industry is completely unregulated & every year some stories appear regarding contaminated and entirely fraudulent supplements (often with the ingredients like soy and wheat that can be actively detrimental).

There're 3 principles to supplementing carefully:
Have nutrients from the food when it is possible.

Human beings are actually adapted to get nutrients that are in whole foods. Many nutrients need organic mineral-activators, enzymes, and synergistic co-factors to be absorbed in a proper way. Whilst they're present in the foods naturally, they're sometimes not there in the isolated nutrients and synthetic vitamins.

A study revealed that an animal or person consuming a diet that consists solely of the purified nutrients in the Dietary Reference Intake, without any benefit of some coordination inherent in the food, might not thrive & probably will not have good health. It argues for supremacy of the food over supplementation in meeting the nutritional needs of people.

The study revealed the risks of reductionist thinking that's typical in the nutritional supplementation and conventional medicine. Rather, people should consider the significance of what they actually call "food synergy":

The important concept about food synergy is depending on the proposition which interrelations between the food constituents are important. The importance is relying on the balance that is between the constituents within your food, how nicely constituents survive the digestion, & the limit to which these appear active at the cellular level.

The study also provides evidence that the whole foods are quite effective as compared to supplements in fulfilling the nutrient requirements:

- Tomato intake has a huge effect on the human prostate tissue rather than the equal amount of lycopene.
- Broccoli as well as whole pomegranates had more antiproliferative & in the effects of vitro chemical than did a few individual constituents.

- Free radicals were decreased by the intake of brassica veggies, independent of the micronutrient mix.

Get nutrients in Naturally Occurring Kind when possible

Isolated and synthetic nutrients do not have similar impacts on your body. This matters whether these nutrients have been created via biological or technologic processes, as the industrial processing often creates a completely new compound along with some other physiological actions. The trans fats that are produced in the ruminant animals (that is conjugated linoleic acids in the dairy items) are good for health, whereas these fats developed in the industrial seed oils processing are quite toxic as well.

Folic acid is one more example. Naturally occurring kind of the folate isn't folic acid, the compound that is not usually found in nature or food, but tetrahydrofolate. Whilst folic acid is converted into the folate, this conversion is not good in human beings. It is also vital to learn that contrary to natural folate, the folic acid doesn't cross placenta. It is important as folate is a very crucial nutrient for the pregnancy, & whilst folic acid could prevent defects in a neural tube it does not have other good effects of the folate. What is more, many studies reveal that folic acid – and not natural folate – does increase the risk of cancer risk. Unluckily, folic acid is what is sometimes used in the multivitamins, as it is not costly than the natural folate.

Be Choosy with Your Supplements.

As, you know that multivitamins are becoming popular so half of the world population is currently taking one. However is it a good thing? Many studies found that these multivitamins either give no advantage or might even do harm. One study was conducted in the "Archives of Internal Medicine" revealed that they have less to no impact on the risks of general cancers, mortality in the postmenopausal females or CVD. An unpopular meta-analysis showed that treatment along with the synthetic beta carotene, vitamins E and A might enhance mortality.

The main issue with the multivitamins is they have just a bit of good nutrients including magnesium, vitamin K2, and vitamin D, & a huge amount of toxic nutrients such as vitamin E, folic acid, iron, and calcium. It means that they can cause some nutrient imbalances which contribute to diseases. One more issue is that manufacturers of multivitamin sometimes use cheap ingredients, like folic acid rather than natural folate.

Recommendations of Lifestyle

The paleo diet is becoming quite common as many people are following the paleo lifestyle. Paleolithic, or paleo, is also known as "Ancestral", "Grain-Free," Whole Food," or "Primal," however, its name is less vital than its principles for having a good and healthy lifestyle. Its main idea is we consume what our previous generations consumed. You might say, "did not people die is they were thirty or forty though?" Its answer is yeah. While you take into account the risks to their lives, like absence of the modern medicine (required in emergency times), predatory animals, infectious disease (even without any help of modern medicine and knowledge), and factors of nature together with insufficient shelter, it is very easy to find how our ancestors' life span was shorter. What is important to know if they weren't experiencing serious lifestyle diseases that millions of people are suffering from these days.

These simple steps would help in forming a solid base for a good lifestyle!

Tips for Paleo diet and lifestyle in general

A paleo diet is reported to free you from migraine, remove bloating, eliminate seasonal allergies, clear up your acne, & help you in shedding some pounds. Whilst none of it's guaranteed, cleaning up the diet & focusing on fresh and whole foods is a good notion. Real foods in appropriate portions assist you in feeling quite satisfied as they aid to keep the levels of blood sugar even & the hunger hormones quite balanced.

The main paleo for the starters guidelines—skip all grains (both whole and refined), dairy, packaged snacks, legumes, & sugar in favor of veggies, fruits, meats, eggs, seafood, nuts, fats, seeds, & oils—sound easy, however, to go successfully a cavewoman takes savvy (Going a caveman is different as compared to following ketosis). You can follow these paleo diet principles for starters.

Pinpoint Motivation

Most individuals turn to the paleo diet in order to assist with medical problems, like GI issues, allergies, and autoimmune conditions as well. Some just have to feel good day-to-day or they believe that it is a healthy way to have food. Your main reason would help you in determining the guidelines that you follow & about what you need to be meticulous. Also, be strict regarding your personal principles for the very first month. It's enough time to begin noticing good changes in your health.

Clean Out Kitchen

Collect all "no" food items on a paleo diet list such as packaged foods, grains, milk, cereal, cheese, vegetable oils, yogurt, and beans, you get this—& toss these in the dust bin. Doing this all has one advantage that is it is easy to avoid the temptation when it is not there at all.

But in case you like to take little steps at first then it does work as well. Probably you can cut dairy items out during the first week, remove refined grains in the second week, skip the grains during the third week, & so on until you are following the paleo diet. In each way, make sure to buy whole foods hence you have got plenty to work with for designing the paleo diet meal plan.

Follow 85/15 Approach

After 1st 30 days, several experts suggest the 85/15 rule, means 85% of the time you are strictly following the paleo diet, leaving 15% for the non-paleo, whether that is one granola bar (that you could opt for the paleo granola recipe), one hamburger (bun & all) at the cookout, or some cocktails. Focus how you actually feel after introducing new things into the paleo diet. For instance, when you have one scoop of yummy ice cream & wake up bloating the next morning, you might decide future discomfort is not worth this.

Cook

As, the paleo diet is based on fresh and whole foods so it is easy to whip meals up at home than the restaurant where it is hard to control what kind of ingredients are there. So, take this golden opportunity to do experiment with the new foods—might be a bit challenging for you to purchase weird-looking veggies at the market & ask the shopkeeper for a piece of advice on how perfectly to cook it. You could search online too or just invest in the paleo diet cookbook for the inspiration hence the meals stay yummy & are not just plain chicken breast along with plain carrots and kale.

Expect 1 Setback (or 2)

It is absolutely normal to follow the paleo diet & slip back into the usual eating habits. But you need not to worry about failure. It is a good learning process. You can also search like-minded people who are already following this diet via local forums, groups, blogs, & Facebook, & connect with those in order to take assistance to keep you on the track—& keep you over there.

The Label Decoder

As, you know to not eat doughnuts, crackers, and cookies, but a few foods are actually not paleo: nut butters, peanut butter (this is a legume); dried fruit along with the added sugars; & lunchmeats, malt vinegar, soy sauce, and other sauces and marinades (some consist of sugar, soy, preservatives, and gluten). Hence make sure to see all ingredients list while purchasing anything in the package.

Think About Your Plate

You are taught to always reserve half plate with vegetables, one quarter for the lean protein, & a remaining quarter for the whole grains. While you actually change to the paleo diet, stop holding some place for the grains: The balanced plate contains a palm-sized protein, one dollop of fats, & vegetables, vegetables, vegetables (fill remaining plate along with these).

Change Your Oil

Rather than reaching for the corn, canola, or soybean oil for frying, you will have to use the lard or coconut oil. Really. Yes, these good-quality saturated fats are good to prepare food with as they are stable

& will not oxidize while heated through (oxidation also releases detrimental free radicals). Also, when this comes to the lard, animal fats—in case, from the grass-fed cows—packed with huge amounts of omega 3, as well as one form of fat known as conjugated linoleic acid that some studies find might help you in burning fat. Some dietitians also suggest butter from the grass-fed cows; however, many restrict the dairy of all kinds. (The choice is all yours.) For the cold applications, you can use walnut oil, olive oil, and avocado oil.

Eat Meat

There are a lot of people who have restricted the meat from the paleo diet as they believe that it is detrimental to health. You could also eat meat—only be sure that it is of high quality. Hence, you can say bye to the processed meats that include bologna, hot dogs, and salami. The wild meats such as bison, boar, and elk are a good choice for you, followed by the pasture-fed poultry as well as meats, & lean grain-fed meat must be the last pick. And, for seafood, go for the wild-caught quite often, and low-mercury and sustainable choices are the best.

You can Easily Make Fool Your Sweet Tooth

Removing sugar is one major tough task for several people in the start. In case, you love to eat a treat right after your dinner then you can swap your cookies or just fro-yo for one piece of the fruit. (For your sugar cravings, experts say that the paleo diet allows dried mangoes.) With the time, the taste buds would adjust accordingly— & that the Oreos that you loved a lot before may become so much sweet for you now. Seriously, it can happen!

You can Eat Out

Some business dinner and brunch with the best friends is possible on a paleo diet. All this takes is just a bit ingredient sleuthing. You need to first look at your menu before time & pick 1 to 2 options which you could paleo-ize. This can be a wild salmon and broccoli. (Also request double the vegetables rather than the rice pilaf.) Also, at a restaurant, do not be ashamed to ask relevant questions regarding the things that are prepared & request alterations, if important.

Eat the Whole Foods which are Nutrient Rich

In case, food isn't in such state that this was while pulled from the soil then there are great chances that it has been refined & is not optimal. By selecting food right from nature, this gives our bodies those nutrients that are required to heal our bodies.

Avoid Nutrient-Poor, Processed, and Refined Foods which are Made in the Factory

It means that the pasteurized dairy, grains, seed oils (canola, cottonseed, corn, and soybean), artificial sweeteners, & refined sugar (fructose corn syrup). Most of these food items rob many nutrients from the body for digestion that negates the basic aim of eating that must be for fueling a human body along with nutrients for growing and repairing itself.

Yeah, it would take some time to learn to paleo lifestyle. There might be some confusion in the start whilst you are working to change the grocery shopping habits, choices of eating outside, and meal preparation, hence this is definitely vital to alter at a gradual pace which suits you perfectly. Plus, know that the most "non-paleo" foods have to be actually re-worked in order to fit the paleo lifestyle.

Eat For Healthy Digestive System

The gut/brain health is of utmost importance for the overall health. For being successful, you have to focus on the signs that the body is actually giving you. In case, you come to know that consuming dairy causes some digestive upset then it's the way your body of telling you about avoiding such food items! Keeping your food log & journal could aid you in spotting latest trends in food consumption & signs. Digestive health is more crucial than many people think. Do you know 60 to 80 percent of the immune system begins in the gut? In case, you are continuously stressing the digestion with some irritating foods then the immune system would be suppressed & your health would suffer a lot.

Eat Food to Keep Steady Blood Sugar

Have you ever felt weak or shaky between your meals? Do you have some kind of swings in the energy level? Chances are, the blood sugar is actually spiking & dropping due to the meals. If you eat sugar and white flour then the blood sugar will spike up & you will feel the rush of energy. While the sugar is managed automatically by the body, your blood sugar also drops & you start to feel like hungry and lethargic. Consuming whole foods would give the body with carbs, enough of proteins, and an ample amount of fats. The combination would let your blood sugar rise even more slowly after having meals & staying elevated between your meals.

As the paleo diet is all about consuming whole foods so it might be good for everybody. The main thing is that this could be easily customized to fit anybody. By keeping one journal about how do you feel throughout the day might make the whole process work smoothly.

First, ask yourself a question of how you feel. Following are a nice starting point:

- When does the energy level fluctuate?
- Do you feel 2 to 3 bowel movements per day?
- What are moods like?
- Do you crave specific foods?

In case not, then you'll benefit from the paleo diet. You can include more veggies in the current paleo food diet; replace the refined grains with the whole grain. And, the success that you actually feel when making these alterations is surely to be somewhat encouraging to keep you continue. Also, before long, you'll have removed nutrient-robbing foods & be filling up along with yummy whole foods!

Whole Foods Intake

Many people have wrong assumptions regarding the truth about the paleo lifestyle. As in reality, this comes down to consuming the whole food. Following are some examples:

- Eggs, meat, and seafood – ideally pasture-raised, grass-fed, organic-fed animals
- Fruits and vegetables– ideally locally grown organic

Some general tips are:
- Make sure to eat veggies at different time periods during your paleo transition because you would find all taste buds alter while your intake changes. And, people who do not like vegetables might find that they encourage their natural salty taste or sweetness while their palate does adapt to the real food.
- You need to be careful to not over-eat fruits as it could be tough on the blood sugar. Try to have two times as many vegetables as fruits.
- Consume seeds and nuts – They are perfect snacks when you are transitioning into the paleo diet. Be conscious of the portion sizes because large amounts might be tough on the gut.
- Oils and fats– Fats are normally used for important body functions. Do a favor to yourself & purchase healthy fats; they're worth more money!

Remove Refined Foods

Whilst paleo rules encourage consuming whole foods, one large aspect about it is the removal of refined foods. It's strongly recommended to remove:
- Whole grains – corn, quinoa, wheat, rice, rye, & some other whole grains are quite healthy. Plus, they can rob a body

having nutrients to be actually digested, & do spikes in the blood sugar.

- Dairy – processed, yogurt, pasteurized milk, and cheese. Raw dairy items are also acceptable for a few people.
- Sweeteners – not each sweetener is created equally. And, natural sugars must be eaten in smaller amounts and manufactured sweeteners must be entirely avoided.
- Refined grains – Such as cereals, pasta, oatmeal, bread, muffins – basically, something made with the white flour.
- Packaged snacks – consists of processed fats, refined grains, and sugars which would be not good for the health.
- Some beverages – remove all artificial drinks and sweeteners that are made with the sugar. And, minimize alcohol and caffeine consumption.

Paleo diet Outside Home

How to Consume Paleo Food Outside Road

Definitely, paleo could be easier in case you are at your home the whole day, but what if you are traveling outside?

In case, you are on vacation, the road warrior, or just going on the cross-country trip with your friends, this might be difficult to eat the paleo food on the road. Also, you do not have always easy access to the grill, & you cannot always plan meals ahead. It might be difficult to consume healthy food & remain paleo.

Do not worry! You can yet eat your paleo food while outside your home. Here is how.

Be Ready

The most vital thing when attempting to have paleo food outside your home is to be ready. Set up yourself for the success from start & plan before time. Know where and when your main pitfalls would come hence that you might plan in order to avoid those.

Remember, the paleo is not "normal" for most individuals. In case, you go for the "business as usual" theory, it will not happen. You would be sucked into everybody else's worse habits. When you have to eat the paleo outside your home, you are about to have to cook yourself & make the diet a priority.

You Should Aim for 80 percent

Firstly, when you are traveling, cut some slack yourself. You might not be 100 percent perfect (as you may be, but this will be difficult). Being outside your home is quite tough hence do not worry about when you actually mess up while trying to consume paleo food on the road. You must have an aim to have paleo 80 percent of the time. The missed meal or some poor snack choice will not kill you. Simply do not let this become a permanent habit.

Rather than attempting to be 110 percent paleo whilst dealing with the continental breakfasts, road trips, client dinners, and conference parties aim to have paleo food on the road 80 percent of the time.

Breakfast

You need to find a dirty diner, & grab some eggs and bacon. Yummy! Yummy! Yummy! When you do not want typical eggs and bacon then you can grab some ingredients and throw those into the omelet, & you are good.

When you are offered potatoes, pancakes, or toast, sub these out for a fruit cup or some bananas instead.

For the morning drink, you can skip the OJ, & have black coffee. This would surely wake you up. In case, you are feeling not good then you might see when they will make this bulletproof.

Next Level Hotels or Restaurants

When you are eating out then it is probably very easy to select your approach just according to the kinds of restaurants that you are going to. A piece of good advice is just to look for a paleo-friendly entree, & order fruits or veggies (preferably).

Mexican

This kind of food is generally quite paleo-friendly when you might avoid the chips and tortillas. A very good paleo Mexican food is fajitas as you might just eat the veggies & meat the tray off, & give tortillas to the friends.

Sushi

It is a nice choice as well. Whilst rice is not strictly paleo, there're surely worse choices. You need to note that sushi rice also contains traces of sugar hence do not stuff your stomach with this, but it is acceptable in a small amount. As the side benefit, along with sushi, you are about to stock up on the Omega-3 with the fresh seafood. When you need to go completely raw as well as avoid the rice completely, grab sashimi.

Seafood

It is paleo-friendly so you can simply eat this up.

American Fare

You'd do very well at such restaurants when you avoid buns, fries, and chips. And, generally serving sources of high-quality meat as compared to most places, all these restaurants typically have veggies as sides, & you could get one solid burger (along with a bun on the side) or some other meat choice along with the side of fruit or veggies.

Steakhouses

In case. You are entertaining your clients then just head to the steakhouse. And, not only you will impress the clients, but also you will eat some amazing paleo food. Everything in the steakhouses is paleo-friendly. Be careful along with the gourmet mac & cheese, mashed potatoes, & other sides that they usually bring out.

You need to skip these sides, pay attention to the entrees, & you will have more. Or, when you are feeling fancy then just check out the all-you-can-eat Brazilian steakhouses & chow down meat.

Italian

You should stay away from this kind of food. If this is not an option then get meatballs or chicken, & try to get killer Caesar salad. Avoid pasta porn. It isn't worth this.

Appetizers and Sides

You might always substitute your fries for the fresh salad. So, take benefit of such an option.

Road Trip

When you are going on the road and driving for many hours then do prep work, & bring one cooler.

Snacks

- Dark chocolate – Try to find some stuff that is 80 percent

- cacao or even higher. Eat this in a smaller amount.
- Beef jerky – It might be a nice snack too, though this could be costly when you select this as your main snack.
- Nuts – Almonds, cashews, walnuts, & much more.
- Trail mix – It is also a nice pre-packaged pick for the paleo snack. You can watch for the mixes out that have tons of peanuts or sweets (peanuts aren't technically paleo-friendly).

Fruits

They must be your favorite desserts outside your home. Be sure that you stock fruit up whenever you can. The following are healthy options:

- Oranges
- Berries (Blueberries, Blackberries, and Raspberries)
- Apples
- Banana (Self-contained food item)

When you need something easy to eat then buy some dried fruits from a grocery store. They are yummy and simple to eat without any juice or mess. Be careful about the high fructose content! Treat them as desserts than as your main dish.

Veggies

Veggies are actually portable snacks. Only wash those and you can eat them. You might easily eat them while you are in a car or on a road. Following are some favorite vegetables (most of these you could try even raw):

- Broccoli (yeah, you might eat it raw)

- Carrots
- Avocado is portable, easy, & tastes delicious.
- Spinach
- Celery

Do Grocery Shopping

It is strange as we discount this, however, you might do grocery shopping when on vacation. It is true! This significantly enhances your ability to consume paleo while outside your home.

If it can be tough to make a meal in case you do not have a kitchen in the hotel room then you would be able to find some prepared or fresh food at some grocery store. A few stores would even make a cut of the meat for you.

When you are driving then you could grab your cooler, & put food. Your cooler would make able you to enjoy a portable and fresh "produce section" in the car to dip into while other good food is not available.

Also, you could get the precooked chicken sausage or whole chicken, & eat it. Or you might stop by a lunch buffet at the grocery store, & eat paleo-friendly from there.

The whole foods buffet is a very good example of it if it is lunchtime.

Paleo Hacks Fast Food

While fast food is a type of the "last resort" then believe this or not, it is possible to actually hack the fast food for making this more paleo-friendly. Here is how you might do it.

Salads

When you start with the base salad then it is really tough to go wrong. And, the best part is that most places give salads nowadays. McDonald's has these as well now (though we do not recommend you McDonald's as the first choice).

Surely, salads do not contain a lot of calories hence feel free to put some chicken, steak, avocado, or other paleo toppings just before you are about to dig in.

It is worth to note that the salad does not need to be some pansy meal which does leave you starving. In reality, it could be exactly opposite to it.

When you do select a salad then look for the salad dressings which contain sugar and HFCS. Ask for the salad without any dressing, or along with dressing, and do not drown the salad.

Burgers without Buns

The easiest paleo meal is to choose to eat one burger without any bun. There are a lot of fast food restaurants which likely to have high-quality meat, & are very good choices to eat paleo food outside your home. Some would even have it as the option on their menu cards. For instance, if you are outside your home at the fast food restaurant, ask for the "Flying Dutchman".

More Fast Food Paleo Hacks

- You might "hack" fast food to make this paleo-friendly.
- In case, you are searching for a restaurant, you might come

- across those restaurants that mark the food as "paleo." When you are fortunate enough to see the one then take advantage of this.
- Panera has the "secret" paleo-friendly menu.
- You can also ask to sub out the normal wheat wraps for the spinach wrap. Also, you might swap out one bun for the lettuce wrap, though often it is simpler to just eat your wrap without the bun.
- You could grab the burrito bowl, & be almost entirely paleo. When you want the protein fix then you can ask for the double meat bowl, & get the eat on!

Myths about a Paleo Diet

There're so many misconceptions regarding the paleo that are essential to dispel! As, there are a lot of people who assume that it is a meat diet or there're so many food items which should be avoided during the Paleo diet. Let me clear up these tiny but serious things!

1. Paleo is way too restricted

There is not just a paleo diet, as people can make different assumptions regarding what this term does mean for them. As many experts say that the paleo diet is just one template and not some dietary prescription.

There are a lot of books that are available on the internet about the paleo diet, & each one has the author's suggestion of what it exactly looks like. Following the paleo diet is about following some guidelines, along with the toughest being removing sugar, grains, dairy, and legumes which mimics how the ancestors used to eat many centuries ago. Most others also advocate the paleo version, along with the Modern paleo, which advocates exclusion of the dairy and grains for the time to actually determine sensitivities & then including these slowly to check out which can work nicely for you.

2. Paleo is the High Meat Diet

This myth is totally wrong. The paleo diet is all about the high vegetable diet. The paleo diet contains roughly 70 percent veggies. You must be wary about any diet which doesn't advocate you consume almost 70 percent veggies in the diet, barring required dietary modifications relying upon some health conditions. Surely, you are consuming meat on the paleo diet; however, its amount differs around the individual tolerances in 10 to 30 percent range. There are a lot of dietitians who say that you must consume almost about .5 to 1 pound (or .22 to .45 kg) of the meat on a daily basis. Any other animal protein other than this could lead to some health issues and decrease the life span. This must include healthy and fresh red meat once a week at least – of course, it must be grass fed!

3. Paleo is a Low Carb Diet

No, this is not right. By definition, it is the low-carb diet. this might or might not be, relying on the chosen foods. White potatoes, sweet potatoes, starchy fruits, yams, and even winter squash are consumed by the paleo folks who want more carbs for fueling the active lifestyle. In addition, my take on the paleo that is the Modern paleo, & others in this movement also advocate eating the non-gluten grains as well as white rice as far as you can tolerate those.

4. Paleo is a costly diet

The answer to this myth is you pay money for good quality foods or pay for the doctors, medications, & nursing homes as well. U.S. citizens spend a small percentage of income on the food as compared to the most industrialized nations – & bad health as a nation actually reflects choices.

Also, we want to spend money on food in order to salvage the health. You have to think about the nutrient density & buying high-quality dairy, eggs, and meat which cost more. Also, you have what you actually pay for – the pastured eggs may be quite costly but you can get 2 to 3 times and even more nutrition. You will consume a similar amount of calories; however, have exorbitantly more nutrition each bite.

Also, with the real paleo food diet, there're a lot of resources in order to assist you in shopping on the budget. You can save your money by purchasing a pie, bread, ice cream, grain products, and cheese. You can pay half amount of what you will at the Whole Foods by actually getting vegetables at some farmer's market. You can also grow your vegetables. You can join such sources. Go in along with some families in order to buy half the grass-fed pig or cow for as less as 3.50 dollars an lb. or a half kilo.

5. Meat Consumers do not live longer than the Vegetarians

Do the vegetarians live longer than the carnivores? Poorly and early done research reveals that the vegetarians usually live longer as compared to meat consumers. The wrong finding has convinced many people to go vegetarian. The Vegetarian Myth does say that census has proved that the vegetarians do not live longer as compared to the meat consumers, no matter what the research work says. But let have look at the research.

When consuming meat enhances the risk of heart disease, as is typically assumed in every medical community, we may expect low rates in vegetarians and vegans. Previous studies have suggested that it's true, however later; carefully conducted studies reveal that it is not. Many early studies are poorly designed & also subject to some confounding factors. The vegetarians likely to be quite healthy on average as compared to the general public – this boosts the life span as well. It is not because of eliminating meat. Other elements describe longevity, like less drinking and smoking, more exercise, to name a few.

The evidence suggests that any health problems that are associated with the meat-eating might not actually come from meat, but the absence of some other healthy food items. For instance, vegetarians typically eat more fruits, vegetables, & nuts. In reality, the study revealed that obvious health advantages of the vegetarianism are not tied too much with the meat absence, however, to the enhanced consumption of healthy foods.

Higher and newer quality research that has attempted to actually control the confounding lifestyle and diet factors have not found survival benefits in becoming a vegetarian. For instance, one study has compared the mortality rate of individuals who did shopping in the food stores (both omnivores and vegetarians) to individuals in the general public. They revealed that both of the groups in the food store actually lived longer as compared to those in the general public. It suggests that consuming meat as a part of the healthy diet doesn't have similar effects as consuming meat as the major part of an unhealthy diet. The similar findings were also confirmed in the study conducted in England in the year 2003 containing 65,000 subjects. The study didn't observe a huge difference in mortality rate between omnivores and vegetarians.

There are a lot of vegetarian sites as well as books cite studies on the Seventh-day Adventists, several are vegetarians. Most studies have found the vegetarian group to be at less risk of the death that non-vegetarians. And, when all results are put together then vegetarianism doesn't confer benefits in terms of death risk. Also, the overall finding in reviewing the studies reveal that the vegetarianism is attached with the improved longevity.

Vegetarian and vegan diets result in a lot of minerals, vitamins, & nutrient deficiencies that include omega 3 fatty acids, B12, taurine, B6, iron, D, zinc, and iodine. If you are consuming a diet that is full of different antinutrient foods such as legumes as well as grains & suffering from several nutrient deficiencies that are unavoidable on a vegetarian diet then how individuals postulate that the vegetarians live long lives as compared to the meat consumers is just beyond me.

6. Did not Cavemen Just Live to thirty?

There are several articles about the paleo diet claiming that the cavemen just lived up to thirty years. That is actually half right. When some caveman made this past age twenty, he generally lived up to sixty years of age. A major issue with the paleo longevity stats is that they actually factor in the infant mortality. Rates of death were higher for the children under 5. Hence, the average longevity age at thirty several reads about is the average of people who actually died in the infancy & people who naturally died due to old age. Some other elements included inferior shelter, infectious disease, and predatory animals.

Let us face this. Cavemen actually lived a difficult existence. The cavemen worked hard for each morsel of the food that they put in the mouths. Most of the energy was consumed foraging & hunting for the animals that they used to do in the sun the whole day. Cavemen also had to face other tribes as well. They had to bear all seasons without air conditioners and heaters. Life was too much tough that we even cannot imagine. Could you think of living outdoors & living off land throughout your life? No, you cannot.

7. We must live the same as our Paleolithic Ancestors As we are the Same Genetically

Many individuals in the ancestral communities trumpet how the genes are identical to our ancestors hence we must eat and live just like them. While you think about this, it's a bit hilarious that the group of individuals who claim to take the evolutionary approach to life does show little understanding about evolution. Humans & chimps have the same genomes to the tune of about 99.5 percent. A major difference between the chimp and the human being is in the gene expression. Due to 2 species have the same genes doesn't mean they would both survive in the same environment or with the same sources of food. One main mechanism through which the adaptations increase is an alteration in the gene expression that is known as epigenetics. Different lifestyles as well as food choices go off and on various genes.

It will be silly to say that epigenome of modern human beings is similar to their ancestors, given essential changes in food and environment which have occurred from that era. The epigenetic alterations could happen quicker. Several sources of food can create pressure for the genetic changes that could happen quickly than many people think. Like, lactase persistence is one of the alterations which happened within the previous 8000 years. It's pretty fast.

8. We have not adapted to the New Food Products Introduced by the Agriculture

This theory goes like: We have evolved over a million years even without eating the food products that are available after the discovery of agriculture. So, we aren't adapted to the foods. However, it assumes that the species is not adapted to the food as it has never consumed this. And in case, you have a look at this evolutionary record that is wrong. There're so many examples of the evolution where many species were discovered and new sources of foods & survive on those. Like human beings as well as meat. Human beings began eating insects, fruits, and plants. Then they also ate bone marrow from the bones & brains from the skulls & eventually became best hunters and gathers. It altered our physiology. And, after the introduction of meat into the diet, we then went from having a large gut which was nice for fermenting the rough cellulose & carb to the big brain and the small gut better for the animal protein digestion. Hence, this goes even without saying when we actually discover new food items, we can also adapt to those, a few more slowly than the others. That is why many people could bear grains & dairy, whilst others cannot. But there is one more reason for the differences in the food tolerances.

Chris Kresser has made an interesting speech in 2013 at the Ancestral Health Symposium. He stated that the main reason we do not tolerate grains along with other food items that aren't paleo isn't because we cannot digest these, but due to missing an important gut bacteria that is required for the digestion. Several hunter-gatherer cultures that were discovered by Weston A. Money thrived on the diets consisting of dairy, grains, & other food items that were not considered the paleo with no disease virtually. He also revealed that individuals in the Lötschental Valley, Switzerland & the Scottish & Gaelic, all depended on dairy as well as grains as staples in the diet. Definitely, they soaked or fermented the grains – something we aren't doing.

The theory that is obvious in a paleo diet community goes like this: a shift from the hunter-gatherers's lifestyle to agriculture actually led to the increase in diseases & a decreasing rate in health. There is no doubt that it is true, however, the notion that compounds such as gluten, lectins, saponins, & capsaicin in the peppers were actually responsible for such decline is not well supported by this evidence. A huge increase in the chronic inflammatory diseases did not occur for most of the part until last 100 years. Still, the alteration from the hunter-gatherers' lifestyle to agriculture did happen about ten-thousand years ago. Hence, there must be something which can explain this decrease in health. When this was true that lectins and gluten in the grains significantly raised the risk of different diseases, they surely would have done it long ago.

Chris Kresser presented a very good theory. He says that it is quite possible that potentially dangerous compounds in the new foods aren't a serious risk element for the inflammatory disease if the Paleo microbiome – the gut bugs – is yet intact. If our microbiome is deficient or depleted, these foods could become major factors of risk for the inflammatory disease.

To repair our gut flora – the microbiome – isn't as easy as supplementing along with probiotics. The supplementation is good & highly recommended; however, the issue lies in how modern life has destroyed the probiotics. Dysbiosis in the guts has begun with a few females breastfeeding that lays the groundwork for the healthy gut. The main colostrum point, a substance which does come before the breast milk in the 7 days of breastfeeding, is for populating the gut along with good bacteria. We consume so much sugar in childhood that also causes overgrowth in the yeast & the gut bacteria. We also pop antibiotics such as candy at a slight hint of the infection, killing good bacteria. Because of refrigeration, people eat less fermented food items – the preservation way which was necessary for preserving food for many years. The fermented foods contain billions of probiotics which help in maintaining the healthy gut. We're destroying natural gut biodome and health due to these practices & several others, such as we are using antibacterial soaps.

Unsecured from enough probiotics colonies, we also develop autoimmune issues, leaky gut, allergies, food intolerances, and inflammatory conditions such as asthma & the host of diseases. These're the rapid growing subsets of diseases nowadays. They're hidden costs of modern hygiene.

Also, Chris Kresser has told that when we yet had the paleo microbiome intact then we might tolerate the grains & all compounds without any problem just like our current hunter-gatherer friends. It is the main point because this resolves a few obvious conflicts in our ancestral paradigm. This might explain the reason different cultures consumed grains for many years & their health conditions that we are attributing to the grains were actually rare. Surely, our height and health have declined after the grains farming, but it doesn't explain what's happening to health today.

Also, you might also expand the paleo diet. Many individuals who spend their time overhauling the gut bacteria can introduce dairy, grains, or some other non-paleo food items – even though they have had the previous intolerances – & do just nice. This explains why people can tolerate foods with no obvious issues whilst others cannot. Hence, work on the good gut health & thus you would safely enjoy the dairy, grains, & some other foods that aren't paleo diet given you do not have any food intolerances to these for the other reasons.

9. A Paleo Diet Increases Cholesterol

Have you ever heard that the fat does not make you look fat? Eating cholesterol-dense foods don't increase cholesterol in any way. The liver does make 85 percent of the cholesterol irrespective of cholesterol consumption in response to the number of several elements – none of these involve consumption of red meat as well as eggs. Hence, eating sugar and grains are the actual culprits – the foods removed from the paleo diet.

10. Cavemen weren't having any Diseases

Cavemen had different symptoms of heart disease. Remember, there are a lot of diseases that have the genetic component that even cavemen could not escape from. They also carried these diseases just as we do but they lived a far better lifestyle hence they were also less prone to activate the genes. A few diseases have strong genetic components which would be expressed despite how healthy someone lives. Hence, some of the paleo munching cavemen also suffered from cancer; however, it was not very common. Most of the cavemen died due to battle wounds as well as accidents, and a few dropped dead due to heart attacks.

7-day Meal Plan

A Paleo Diet Menu for 7 days for a Woman who wants to Lose Weight

It is a sample menu that consists of a balanced amount of paleo-friendly food items. And, by all means, you can easily adjust this sample menu that relies on your own choices.

Day 1

Breakfast (271 kcal)

- Avocado Egg Toast – 1 serving
- A.M. Snack (42 kcal)
- Blueberries – ½ cup

Lunch (374 kcal)

- Pita Bread and Hummus with Green Salad - 1 serving

P.M. Snack (62 kcal)

- Medium orange - 1

Dinner (457 kcal)

- Green Peppercorn Sauce with Seared Salmon - 1 serving
- Steamed green beans - 1 cup
- Medium red potato (1 baked), drizzled with olive oil (1 tsp.), nonfat plain Greek yogurt 1 Tbsp. and pepper (1 pinch).

Daily Totals: 28 g fiber, 1,296 mg sodium, 1,206 calories, 10 g sat. fat., 62 g protein, 49 g fat, 140 g carbohydrates

Day 2

Vegetable-Hummus Sandwich

Breakfast (287 kcal)

- Bran cereal - 1 cup
- Skim milk - 1 cup
- Blueberries - 1/2 cup

A.M. Snack (95 kcal)

- Medium apple - 1

Lunch (325 kcal)

- Vegetable-Hummus Sandwich - 1 serving

P.M. Snack (80 kcal)

- Medium and sliced red bell pepper - 3/4
- Hummus - 2 Tbsp.

Dinner (426 kcal)

- Peanut Noodle Salad and Roasted Tofu - 2 cups

Daily Totals: 1,324 mg sodium, 1,212 calories, 6 g sat. fat., 55 g protein, 42 g fat, 48 g fiber, 183 g carbohydrates

Day 3

Avocado-Lime Dressing with Grilled Romaine

Breakfast (276 kcal)

- Nonfat plain Greek yogurt - 1 cup
- Blueberries - 1/2 cup
- Slivered almonds - 1 1/2 Tbsp.

- Honey - 2 tsp.
- Top yogurt with honey, blueberries, and almonds

A.M. Snack (102 kcal)
- Medium carrots - 2
- Hummus - 2 Tbsp.

Lunch (320 kcal)
- Peanut Noodle Salad and Roasted Tofu - 1 1/2 cups

P.M. Snack (46 kcal)
- Strawberries - 1 cup

Dinner (460 kcal)
- Avocado-Lime Dressing and Grilled Romaine - 1 serving
- Paprika-Herb Chicken Rubbed - 1 serving
- cooked quinoa with olive oil (1 tsp.) and salt (1 pinch) - 1 cup

Daily Totals: 1,263 mg sodium, 1,204 calories, 6 g sat. fat., 79 g protein, 42 g fat, 26 g fiber, 135 g carbohydrates.

Day 4

Tomato Cream Sauce with Cod
Breakfast (265 kcal)
- Bran cereal - 1 cup
- Skim milk - 3/4 cup
- Blueberries - 1/2 cup

A.M. Snack (95 kcal)

- Medium apple - 1

Lunch (374 kcal)
- Pita Bread and Hummus with Green Salad - 1 serving

P.M. Snack (62 kcal)
- Medium orange - 1

Dinner (407 kcal)
- Tomato Cream Sauce with Cod - 1 serving
- Brown rice cooked - 1/2 cup
- 1 teaspoon olive oil with steamed broccoli tossed - 1 cup

Daily Totals: 1,370 mg sodium, 1,202 calories, 8 g sat. fat., 54 g protein, 34 g fat, 43 g fiber, 195 g carbohydrates,

Day 5

Fried Rice Chicken Cauliflower Breakfast (293 cal)
- Rolled oats (1/2 cup) cooked in one cup milk
- Sliced strawberries - 1/2 cup
- Cook oats & top with cinnamon (1 pinch) and strawberries.

A.M. Snack (90 kcal)
- Sliced bell pepper - 1/2
- Hummus - 3 Tbsp.

Lunch (350 kcal)
- Loaded Nacho Black Bean Soup - 1 serving

P.M. Snack (84 kcal)

- Blueberries - 1 cup

Dinner (304 kcal)

- Cauliflower Chicken Fried "Rice" - 1 1/4 cups

P.M. Snack (92 kcal)

- Kiwi and Mango with Lime Zest - 3/4 cup

Daily Totals: 31 g fiber, 1,170 mg sodium, 1,214 calories, 8 g sat. fat., 62 g protein, 42 g fat, 161 g carbohydrates

Day 6

Tostada Toaster-Oven
Breakfast (328 kcal)

- Bran cereal - 1 cup
- Skim milk - 1 cup
- Blueberries - 1 cup

A.M. Snack (62 kcal)

- Medium orange - 1

Lunch (296 kcal)

- Tuna with Dill Salad and White Bean - 1 serving
- P.M. Snack (46 kcal)
- Strawberries - 1 cup
- Dinner (457 kcal)
- Tostada Toaster-Oven - 1 serving

Daily Totals: 1,203 mg sodium, 1,188 calories, 8 g sat. fat., 55 g protein, 39 g fat, 49 g fiber, 184 g carbohydrates

Day 7

Skillet Chicken Lemon & Kale with Potatoes

Breakfast (355 kcal)

- Egg Avocado Toast - 1 serving
- Blueberries - 1 cup
- A.M. Snack (46 kcal)
- Strawberries - 1 cup
- Lunch (372 kcal)
- Tuna, Dill Salad and White Bean - 1 serving
- Toasted whole-wheat bread, toasted - 1 slice

P.M. Snack (62 kcal)

- Medium orange - 1

Dinner (374 kcal)

- Skillet Chicken (200 g) Lemon and Kale with Potatoes (200 g) - 1 serving

Daily Totals: 27 g fiber, 1,289 mg sodium, 1,209 calories, 9 g sat. fat., 64 g protein, 50 g fat, 130 g carbohydrates

There's typically no need for tracking macronutrients and calories (such as protein, fat or carbs) on a paleo diet, never in the start.

But, if you want to lose tons of weight then it's a nice notion to cut carbohydrates somewhat & limit the consumption of high-fat foods like nuts.

1200 Calories Day Meal Plan for a Man

Summary

As a Paleo diet does involve cutting on the processed foods down, it is definitely a nice way to avoid the junk. It is a caveman diet that bans calorific processed foods high-fat, booze, & refined carbohydrates (though the diet fizzy liquids are not prohibited).

This encourages people to consume more high-quality protein that includes lean meat, fish, and chicken that helps in keeping you full for the whole day. Consuming more vegetables, nuts, and fruits is a healthy way to increase fiber & to assist in filling you up & to boost intake of antioxidants, vitamins, and minerals.

But, there're many concerns attached to the caveman diet. As dairy items are removed, intake of the bone-building calcium is quite low, & the lack of exercise would not assist you in toning and strengthening your body. But these are not right as literature has proved this.

Most people who follow a Paleo Diet feel healthy. They also lose their weight by decreasing the consumption of fats. Combined with different reports of good health, no migraines, and fewer diseases you need to think about the Paleo diet as it is very good.

Like major changes in lifestyle and diets, if you follow this diet then first ease yourself into this slowly. With the same meal plans, there is no need of adopting any extreme way for faster results. Your approach must be to change and modify depending on your lifestyle and needs.

Made in the USA
Middletown, DE
09 September 2019